*John D. Allen, MS*

# Gay, Lesbian, Bisexual, and Transgender People with Developmental Disabilities and Mental Retardation
## Stories of the Rainbow Support Group

*Pre-publication REVIEWS, COMMENTARIES, EVALUATIONS . . .*

"John Allen's journalistic skill helps the reader understand the complexity of social and sexual interaction among GLBT people who have been labeled DD/MR. This is a much-needed text of hope and change in a domain that needs greater humanity. The human services designed to improve the quality of life of this population are too often characterized as socially conservative and moralistic. These values are translated into social interventions that often fail to recognize the full range of psychosexual needs of clients. Developmental disabilities is a service area in which clients are too often treated as children, and as result, heterosexuality is ignored and homosexuality is oppressed.

The focus of this book, the Rainbow Support Group, is designed to assist clients through the coming-out process, to explore their homosexuality, and to develop safe and satisfying same-sex relationships. The group includes a variety of modalities and is the first of its kind. Anecdotal evidence shows this group to be an effective human service intervention for the GLBT population.

Allen uses personal narratives of members of the RSG to uncover the pain and joy of sexual discovery and self-realization. This is more a documentary of the struggle of GLBT people with developmental disabilities than a theoretical analysis. It is a text that helps us to understand how the members of this group act on their desires for companionship, intimacy, and healthy sexual expression."

**George Appleby, DSW, LCSW**
Interim Dean, School of Health and Human Services, and Professor of Social Work, Southern Connecticut State University, New Haven

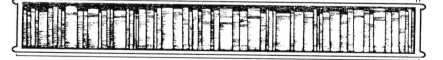

"John Allen and the members of the Rainbow Support Group proudly enlighten us about a safe place for men and women with intellectual disabilities who are GLBT and questioning adults with intellectual disabilities to find understanding, support, and sometimes even friendship.

In their own words, RSG members tell their stories, simply and without self-pity. Some are self-assured, some are shy, but all have the courage to be known, and in that, courage to help other men and women to do the same. These are biographies that have been untold and these men and women have been silent for too long. Now they have a voice: their own!"

**Leslie Walker-Hirsch, MEd**
Social Development and Sexuality
Consultant, Moonstone Sexuality
Education and Consultation Services

❧

"John Allen's sensitivity and joy in working with people with disabilities comes through in his writing, which takes a much-needed and compassionate look at a timely and sometimes difficult subject. Throughout his career, John has been at the forefront of the fight for civil rights for people with disabilities, and he continues that effort with this book."

**Diane Smith**
Radio Talk Show Host;
Author, *Absolutely Positively Connecticut*

❧

"On the simplest but very important level, John Allen's book is a vital and compelling tale of activism and grassroots organizing that can literally change lives. To read the stories of these women and men who find community, companionship, support, and love—which in many cases had been actively denied them—is stirring and joyful. The opening of the institutional closet door for people with mental disabilities is a triumph for the GLBT movement and certainly an enactment of its original, inclusive, and liberatory vision.

But Allen's book is much more. As the women and men he writes about here discover a safe, supportive space in which to come out and be themselves, they also discover the depth and the breadth of their own sexual longings and desires. While not about sex per se, this book is a tribute to the enormous power of eroticism in the lives of the RSG members and a testimony to the vitality of the erotic in all of our lives."

**Michael Bronski**
Visiting Scholar, Women's Studies
and Jewish Studies, Dartmouth College;
Author, *Culture Clash: The Making
of Gay Sensibility* and *The Pleasure
Principle: Sex Backlash and the Struggle
for Gay Freedom*

❧

"This is a tremendously valuable book. And its value is not limited to the GLBT community. Anyone involved in any way with people with developmental disabilities and mental retardation will come away educated, inspired, and involved. It is a powerful book for any member of the human race, because all of us come in contact with people who are 'different.' By showing, strongly but compassionately, that every human being is also a sexual being, John Allen encourages us to look beyond our differences and celebrate our commonalities. That is a lesson all of us need desperately to learn."

**Dan Woog**
Author, *School's Out:
The Impact of Gay and Lesbian
Issues on America's Schools*

# Gay, Lesbian, Bisexual, and Transgender People with Developmental Disabilities and Mental Retardation

*Stories of the Rainbow Support Group*

# Gay, Lesbian, Bisexual, and Transgender People with Developmental Disabilities and Mental Retardation
## *Stories of the Rainbow Support Group*

John D. Allen, MS

Harrington Park Press®
An Imprint of The Haworth Press, Inc.
New York • London • Oxford

Published by

Harrington Park Press®, an imprint of The Haworth Press, Inc., 10 Alice Street, Binghamton, NY 13904-1580.

PUBLISHER'S NOTE
In this book, individuals' names are used with their permission. Names have been changed where individuals did not grant permission for their names to be used.

Cover design by Jennifer M. Gaska.

Cover photo: Rainbow Support Group members pose in front of the Stonewall Cafe, Greenwich Village, NYC; the birthplace of the modern gay movement.

**Library of Congress Cataloging-in-Publication Data**

Allen, John D. (John Darrett), 1956-
    Gay, lesbian, bisexual, and transgender people with developmental disabilities and mental retardation : stories of the Rainbow Support Group / John D. Allen.
        p. cm.
Includes bibliographical references.
    ISBN 1-56023-395-8 (hardcover : alk. paper)—ISBN 1-56023-396-6 (softcover : alk. paper)
    1. People with mental disabilities—United States—Sexual behavior. 2. Developmentally disabled—United States—Sexual behavior. 3. Gays—United States. 4. Lesbians—United States. 5. Bisexuals—United States. 6. Transsexuals—United States. 7. Gender identity—United States. 8. Self-help groups—United States—Case studies. I. Rainbow Support Group. II. Title.
    HQ30.5 .A45 2003
    306.7'087'4—dc21
                                                                                    2002015133

To my partner Keith Hyatte

# ABOUT THE AUTHOR

**John D. Allen, MS, BS,** is the Program Director of Employment Services at Marrakech, Inc., a human service agency based in Woodbridge, Connecticut. John received an MS in urban studies and a BS in economics from Southern Connecticut State University in New Haven. He is the founder of the New Haven Gay & Lesbian Community Center and the Rainbow Support Group, and is a member of the National Lesbian and Gay Journalists Association, the Connecticut Critics Circle, and the Connecticut Press Club. John lives in Branford, Connecticut, with his partner Keith Hyatte, the Charge Scenic Artist at Long Wharf Theatre.

# CONTENTS

# SECTION III: THE LEADERS

# Preface

Part of what binds the gay community is an experience known as "coming out," in which a person acknowledges his or her sexual orientation to family and friends. The process of coming out is one that usually occurs over time once an individual develops a comfort level with his or her sexuality (Bernstein, 1995).

Although the process is complicated, it is doubtful that even those who are most understanding can imagine the obstacles of trying to navigate the intricacies of sexual orientation discovery by a person with a developmental disability. Acknowledging that people with mental retardation are sexual is a new development in the human service field, but one that is still facing pre-Stonewall mentality regarding those who are gay. Although people with mental retardation are given unprecedented freedom to make personal vocational decisions, there is an unfounded expectation that they do not have sexuality—let alone homosexuality.

As antiquated institutions are closed and residents are moved into more mainstream settings, some human rights issues have been inadequately addressed. Perhaps it is because of an enduring paternalistic attitude that people with mental retardation are childlike and require protection from adult experiences. Personal biases of support staff and guardian family members also serve to restrict individual freedoms.

With great strides being made in human services, hopefully a new understanding is emerging which recognizes that healthy sexuality is a natural component of being an adult.

The Rainbow Support Group (RSG) is evidence that some people with developmental disabilities are gay, lesbian, bisexual, and transgender (GLBT). Among the first of its kind in the nation, the RSG has been meeting since September 1998 at the New Haven Gay & Lesbian Community Center. Participants discuss the same concerns as other gay people, but they do it in a support system that recognizes their unique perspective.

Discussions at the monthly meetings have a surprisingly familiar sound. Members are concerned with being forced into heterosexual

social situations, since that is the only available option for them to socialize. Some members are afraid of being "outed" to their peers and
staff, which is understandable since many people with disabilities are
not their own legal guardians. They are acutely sensitive to retaliation
from staff and family, such as being ostracized from family functions
or ridiculed by unsupportive staff. Transportation is a significant bar-
rier to participation in the group, since most people with developmental disabilities do not drive; it is most often the reason for missed
meetings.

Members may be reluctant to add another level of stigma by identi-
fying themselves as members of the gay community. However, the
primary concerns members describe involve an overwhelming sense
of isolation, lack of companionship, and lack of support from staff
concerning their sexual orientation.

The RSG is an appropriate avenue for members to connect with
others like themselves and also to connect with the larger New Haven
gay community. So far, members have attended such community center events as holiday parties, movie nights, and gay pride celebrations.

The positive outcomes displayed once an individual enters the
group are exciting. Members quickly develop a sense of ownership
and wear rainbow-emblazoned clothing to meetings. Everyone has
joined the host community center to receive regular mailings and
event discounts.

Supervising staff report that members perform better at work, have
fewer behavioral issues, and experience a greater feeling of content-
ment. For people with mental retardation, the ability to say the words
"gay," "lesbian," "bisexual," and "transgender" in an affirming environment is a cutting-edge breakthrough.

# Acknowledgments

Thanks to Katherine R. Allen—sister, friend, and mentor. This project would not have been possible without your generous assistance.

Thanks to my family for their constant support: Jack and Betty Allen; Beth Darrett; Katherine Allen and Matthew Special; Dan and Nancy Allen and Matthew Correira; Doug Allen and Cory Cullen and Vickey Allen, Meg Allen, and Ned Allen; Jean Routt and Richard Shanahan; Laura Hyatte; Gale and Danny Greenlaw; Lori and Adam Sheeler and Madison Sheeler; Lana Greenlaw; Steve and Ella Jane Taylor and Janelle Taylor; Gary and Shelley Hyatte and Kila Hyatte and Keith D. Hyatte; and in loving memory of Keith and Marcella Hyatte.

Thanks to Maureen Thomas and Judy Tompkins who have generously contributed their time and understanding.

Thanks to all of the Rainbow Support Group members and support staff including Andy, Joe, Ron, Pam, Dana, Steven, Bill, Tim, Ben, Lisa, Daniel, Will, Allen, Bob, Steve, Judy Goldberg, Peter McKnight, Denis Caron, John Lawson, Adrianne Prioleau, the many other people who have participated in the group over the years, and those who wish to remain anonymous.

Thank you to Michael F. Collins, Bruce Knox, and Larry Kramer.

The Rainbow Support Group exists because of the generous support of Marrakech, Inc. of Woodbridge; Easter Seals Goodwill Industries of New Haven; and the State of Connecticut Department of Mental Retardation.

Thanks to Joe Parente, Catherine Shanley, Kathy Woods, Carlene DiBiaso, Silvia Moscariello, Joseph R. Rigoglioso, George Appleby, Suzanne Letso, Sean Flanigan, Marcus Linn, Nancy Peterson, Brenda Mohrland, Marilyn Bergen, and Peggy Arthur for their professional support.

Thanks to the New Haven Gay & Lesbian Community Center staff, members, volunteers, and board of directors, including Tammy Aiello, Betty Bourret, Frank DeMayo, keha esposito, Richard Kiyomoto, Paul Kuehn, Dorothy Perta, Julie Schlessel, David Sirois, Joel Whitten, and Richard Wurtzel.

Thanks to Kathryn duPree and Dimitri Triantafillakis of the State of Connecticut Department of Mental Retardation.

Thanks to Brigitte Greenberg and the Associated Press; Daniel Karslake and In The Life Television; Lauren Incognito, John Sykes, and Metroline Publications; Jeriann Geller and Elm City Publications; Larry Connor and *Bay Windows;* Don Church, Fred Kuhr, and *In Newsweekly;* Angela Carter, Arnold Gold, and the *New Haven Register;* Bill Williams and *The Hartford Courant* for helping to share the message of the Rainbow Support Group.

Thanks to Bill Palmer, Rebecca Browne, and The Haworth Press, Inc.

This book is dedicated to GLBT people with developmental disabilities everywhere in their desire for companionship, intimacy, and healthy sexual expression.

# *SECTION I:*
# *BACKGROUND*

# Chapter 1

# Reflections at Four Years:
# A Brief History
# of the Rainbow Support Group

At the start of an important day, fifteen of us had gathered on May 1, 2002, to speak at a conference on Developmental Disabilities/Mental Retardation (DD/MR). After greeting one another in the great hall of the New Haven Union Train Station for an adventure into New York City and a prestigious international conference, our huddle started moving toward the escalators for the descent to the train platforms. We were excited to see so many members attending and were happy to be able to attend together. This was the group's third visit to the conference to speak about the Rainbow Support Group (RSG), and everyone was excited about rounding out our "gay day" with a quick visit to Greenwich Village. For some members, this would be their first time traveling to New York City, riding on the subway, visiting gay sites in the Village, and speaking in public. The day was off to a great start—we were full of anticipation, the culmination of four years of hard work and camaraderie.

Within steps of the landing, Teddy Kennedy Jr. hurried past our crowd before we clogged the path. Kennedy, a local resident, is the nephew of the founder of the Special Olympics and is himself a person with a physical disability, having lost a leg to cancer as an adolescent. This seemingly insignificant moment was a fleeting reminder of how tenuously the RSG operates within the human services profession and changes the lives of people with disabilities.

How can just one group change the perceptions of a profession and, ultimately, society in general? Our clan crossed paths that morning with a member of the Kennedy clan, whose name is synonymous with the Special Olympics—a movement that forever changed perceptions for people with mental retardation. A celebrity figure known to the world, Kennedy is an accessible local citizen who makes no effort to conceal his disability or hide what makes him different and at the same time unique. Simply through his visibility, the man who passed by us serves as a source of strength for anyone to tap. That is the legacy of the RSG. The more visible this minority within a minority becomes, the easier it is for others to become more visible.

The Rainbow Support Group was not something I set out to create. Rather, it came to me, and I believe it did for a reason. I was in a good position to listen and respond to some of the subtle cues that were surfacing throughout Connecticut.

Connecticut has a history of being more supportive of the sexual minority community than other states in the country (Connecticut Women's Education and Legal Fund [CWELF], 1995). In 1969, it was the second state to repeal sodomy laws that criminalized homosexuality and was the third state in 1991 to offer civil rights protections for gay people (CWELF, 1995). Connecticut has a vibrant gay culture with businesses, institutions, and a visibility that is needed to encourage and support others in their desire to live an openly gay life.

As a long-term community activist and a human services professional, my office must have appeared to be a safe place to seek answers about GLBT people with DD/MR. In addition, as the founder of the New Haven Gay & Lesbian Community Center (NHGLCC), the process to create the center was a public effort that frequently identified me and my employer in newspaper articles and television spotlights. Over a two-year period, I logged more than one dozen statewide telephone calls from staff desperately attempting to respond to the sexual-orientation needs of their clients that through neglect had become crises. After receiving a particularly upsetting telephone call, an idea materialized and a plan of action was implemented.

"Several of us would like to float an idea around the state to see if there is an interest in starting this support group," I remember telling my agency's division leader, Joe Parente, in April 1998. I wanted to use the letterhead of the agency, a respected name throughout Connecticut, for a statewide announcement of the proposed group. His response stunned me.

"We'd like to sponsor this project," said Parente without a moment's pause. "This is considered a human rights issue and [sexual orientation] is something that is not being addressed."

Over the next five months, several planning meetings were held to gain support from agencies and staff, establish guidelines for participation and discussions, and begin educating the profession. Sexuality issues for people with DD/MR are still considered, at best, an off-limits topic (Kempton, 1998). We were faced not only with the challenge of educating staff to acknowledge that clients can have a sexual orientation other than heterosexual but also to acknowledge that clients are entitled to opportunities for privacy, intimacy, and sexual expression.

While the RSG has had a tremendous impact on its members (and we would like to think it has also had an impact on the profession), the activities of the group have changed little since our first meeting at the New Haven Gay & Lesbian Community Center in September 1998. The group has remained consistent both in size and topics of discussion. A core group of eight to ten members regularly attends, but over the years more than two dozen members have connected with the group from around the state. Without question, the early support from a state agency helped provide cover for those clients and staff interested in attending and also helped silence any institutional homophobia that would have inevitably been directed at the group. From the start, the RSG has been deliberate in broadcasting its message to the profession and the general community, which has certainly contributed to its success. If nothing else, the RSG has opened a dialogue to allow clients, staff, and the general community to feel less inhibited about the subject.

## The Group

The RSG has evolved into a support group for gay, lesbian, bisexual, and transgender people with developmental disabilities. All four components of the modern gay movement are represented—gay men, lesbian women, and people who identify themselves as bisexual and transgender.

*Transgender* is an umbrella term that refers to people who cross-dress, including males who wear feminine clothing and females who wear masculine clothing (Gay & Lesbian Alliance Against Defamation [GLAAD], 2001). It also includes people who are in various stages of having gender reassignment surgery or become transsexual (GLAAD, 2001). As an example, the RSG includes a fifty-five-year-old male member who identifies as heterosexual, has a girlfriend, yet has cross-dressed his entire life.

The RSG neither encourages nor discourages relationships between members, but as in any other social group, members are able to develop friendships outside of meetings. As members become more comfortable with one another over time, they have developed friendships outside of the group.

The RSG meets on the second Monday of each month and always holds meetings at the New Haven Gay & Lesbian Community Center. There are several reasons for meeting at the center. As a focal point for gay life in southern Connecticut, the center hosts dozens of social and support groups, publishes a newsletter, maintains a Web site, and produces many events during the year.

The center offers a pleasant and accepting atmosphere, providing members the opportunity to enjoy the nurturing surroundings. For some, time spent at the center is their only gay experience. The center is a clearinghouse for gay literature and periodicals, and has a bulletin board for community postings.

The center is also home to many other groups and activities, which members are free to access on their own. When new members first attend, many display a visible sense of satisfaction, expressing a feeling that, "I've come home. I've found others who think like me. I'm not alone." There are movie nights when current videos are shown on a large screen television, dances, other group parties, and holiday parties. Through the RSG, the center has become more user-friendly for the primary reason that members have developed their own friends and new reasons to visit the center.

### The Issues

If we as a profession believe that people with DD/MR are entitled to make vocational, social, and residential choices, there should also be respect for their decisions for sexually intimate relationships. The Rainbow Support Group has revealed that persons with cognitive disabilities have the intellectual capacity to decipher the intricacies of sexual orientation.

Members who do attend the RSG are able to articulate their feelings and demonstrate that they understand what it means to be part of the sexual minority community. Members come to the group with their own sets of concerns, but they report an overwhelming sense of isolation and loneliness. At the very least, participation in the RSG gives members the opportunity to know other people who have similar feelings.

Topics of conversations vary from mundane to personal to explicit perceptions and events. Just as in any other group, the conversation meanders as the focus moves around the room, but members are always free to speak without censoring their gay perspective. For ninety minutes each month, members can feel liberated, be nurtured by the environment, connect with others like them, and take home literature to carry them through another month.

### Successes

The rainbow is a symbol of gay pride and solidarity (Marcus, 1993). In keeping with the symbol, members named the group during their second meeting to declare their pride as gay people and their solidarity with the gay community.

Among the first of its kind in the nation, the RSG has been deliberately public with its message that some people with DD/MR are gay. The RSG publishes a newsletter that is regularly mailed to several hundred addresses, holds regular monthly meetings, garners significant media coverage, and serves as a hub for countless calls from around the country. Just by continuing to meet, the RSG is able to counter the stigma associated with mental retardation and sexual orientation.

The RSG is generating real change, literally one person at a time. Many members may have no experiences in their life that delineate their gayness, yet they know they have feelings of same-sex attraction. The RSG provides members an opportunity to at least have a shared experience where they can meet other people and learn about the gay community. By participating in the group, members can develop new friendships, attempt to arrange dates, and increase their chances of finding a partner. They can learn about appropriate ways to meet others, learn about safe sex, and feel empowered to advocate for their own intimacy needs.

Although it is not a dating service, members in the RSG have had success forming relationships with one another. Two of the group's lesbian members exchanged e-mail addresses following their first meeting together in February 2001 and by March had declared the start of a relationship. Later that year in November, they moved into their own apartment, supported by a state agency, as an openly lesbian couple. The journey to assist them in their relationship was not without problems, but the same can happen in any relationship.

Other significant outcomes with the group involve several male members and their desire for dating and relationships. From the start, the men hopscotched from one to another, but in retrospect, obtaining a partner seemed secondary to the activity of dating. As happens in many dating situations, it seemed they were more excited when they were in pursuit of a partner than after they declared their mutual consent for a relationship. It was when they were on the cusp of settling into a long-term commitment that the bickering began and they romantically pursued unattainable staff and acquaintances.

Similarly, the group's cross-dressing transgender member endured tremendously difficult periods before he finally found support for his dream, which was to spend much of his leisure time cross-dressing. He was threatened with blackmail, humiliated, manipulated, condemned, proselytized, and ignored, all for what seemed natural to him. Here is a man who works, earns his own money, maintains an apartment, and is his own legal guardian, yet his time and desires were not his own. The RSG was a quiet force that assisted him in connecting with support staff who wanted only to listen to him and not try to force him to conform to someone else's expectations.

What has also surfaced as RSG members speak at conferences around the country is that the human services profession has done little to address the desire of people with DD/MR to have opportunities for intimacy. The RSG has done more than simply advocate for sexual minority people with DD/MR; it has become a catalyst for discussing sexuality of the DD/MR heterosexual majority as well. Sexuality is the elephant in the room, given reliance on government funding and public perception of sexuality as a politically loaded term (Hingsburger, 1991). While many direct care support staff either avoid the topic or are moralistic about sexuality, they also feel frustrated and powerless to assist the people they serve with such an important and deeply private aspect of life (Monat-Haller, 1992). It is exciting and groundbreaking that the RSG is assisting the disabled community in having a discussion on the rights of all individuals to sexual expression.

The RSG is building a framework for what is surely to come later. Its success is the ability of members to live open and honest lives. Sexuality is a natural component of adulthood and to deny someone access to his or her feelings renders that person invisible. Ultimately, the power of the RSG lies in its self-advocacy and declaration of purpose.

## Lessons Learned

The RSG is such a tremendous source of strength for its members and an educational resource for the profession that it seems counterproductive to discuss any of the obstacles to its success. However, the issues raised here serve as a reminder that triumphs rise from adversity.

As founder and a facilitator of the RSG, my name serves as a flash point not only for family members and staff uncomfortable with GLBT issues but also for members and other clients who are grappling with their own sexual orientation. The RSG is a member-driven group in which we talk about whatever is on our minds and try to respond if not with cohesion, then with support. During a particularly difficult period in the group, when we were waiting for a national television feature to air on public broadcasting stations, several family members and staff had a typical reaction to our very public "outing." When gay people come out of the closet, very often their family members have the opposite reaction and go into the closet (Bernstein, 1995).

Some of the members who attend RSG meetings are their own legal guardians and have the legal right to make their own decisions. Still, that does not preclude concerned family members from getting involved in their decisions.

The RSG is a controversial group because it deals with the subject of sexuality in the DD/MR community, which is taboo. For example, the father of an RSG member was aware his adult child was attending the group, but took umbrage at some of the publicity surrounding the television feature and the fact his child was prominently featured.

"If you were truly interested in helping them, you would do it quietly and not celebrate [homosexuality]," said this father, suggesting that I had coerced members to appear on television.

As a human services professional obligated to listen to the messages of my clients, my response was that the group was at risk of losing its momentum without publicity in the general community to help normalize the subject. "The best way to make life better for the members is to celebrate who they are," I said.

It is difficult to take an in-between stance when it comes to celebrating who you are. Can you be a little bit gay? How do you make a quiet public announcement about a unique group in a local community? A public message is just that—public—and since there is so much anxiety surrounding the sexuality of people with DD/MR, many people feel that a public dialogue on the subject should be introduced gradually, if at all.

The most courageous person during this episode was the RSG member. At the meeting following the exchange with his parent, the member said to another member (who was also going through a similar experience with family members), "Stick up for your rights. I did."

Statistically, 3 percent of the American population experiences mental retardation (The Arc, 1982). If 10 percent of those 7.5 million Americans are members of the GLBT community, there is much work to do to provide support in the human services profession. Even if the numbers are only 1 or 2 percent, service providers still need to put aside their personal biases toward sexuality and sexual orientation to assist the people they serve. So the question becomes, What is the best way to reach those people about the message of the RSG?

There is a dilemma in trying to broadcast the message of a controversial subject. If the message is too blatant, it offends many conservative stakeholders; but if it is too vague, the message is easily ignored or fails to generate interest. Trying to find the right balance in disseminating information on the RSG has been a source of many of the battles we have faced.

As a unique group, part of the strategy for validating the RSG has been to entrench the group in institutional and professional structures. Although the media has been one of the legs of support, forging formal and informal links with human services and gay community organizations has also contributed to maintaining a viable group. Creating a network of contacts has increased the likelihood that the group will be considered for referrals, welcomed at gay events, and invited to professional conferences. Once again, the approach creates a more visible group, which can challenge the comfort level of even the staunchest supporter.

One of the more proactive administrators at an agency that has consistently demonstrated its support for the RSG and for acknowledging the sexuality of its clients was faced with such a scenario. In preparation for an awards ceremony, I had nominated several individuals and organizations for their support of the RSG. The award was the Jane Addams Award (Jane Addams was the founder of the social work movement) for institutional courage from the Connecticut Coalition for LGBT Civil Rights—a prestigious gay community organization dedicated to civil rights. The group is modeled after other civil rights organizations such as the National Association for the Advancement of Colored People (NAACP) and the Anti-Defamation League (ADL).

After submitting a lengthy application and sharing copies with key players, the administrator called to say the nomination had breached a confidence and must be rescinded immediately. His primary concerns were that the town where his agency was located was a working-class community in which gay issues were not part of the local dialogue. The board of directors for his agency was also unaware of the quiet support that had been offered.

During a follow-up meeting in which we both had a more relaxed opportunity to explain our actions, the crux of the dilemma was revealed. A new organization needs to generate awareness and credentials as it attempts to build a network. For the administrator, the reaction exemplified the internalized homophobia we all must overcome to fully embrace the message of the RSG.

"Would you have had the same reaction if you were nominated for a Jane Addams Award from the NAACP? Would you have declined to accept a Jane Addams Award from the ADL?" I asked, without expecting or receiving a reply.

Similarly, at a statewide conference on DD/MR where the RSG was invited to present a seminar, a description of the RSG was sent beforehand for publication in a conference guide. The description was edited, without permission or notification, which created great confusion for some attendees who expected something else once the presentation began.

The submitted description follows:

> The RSG provides a safe space for discussion and fellowship among people with developmental disabilities who are gay, lesbian, bisexual, and transgender. This emerging issue, along with sexuality and relationships, will be discussed.

The edited description, however, appeared as such:

> The RSG provides a safe space for discussion and fellowship among people with developmental disabilities who have alternative lifestyles. This emerging issue, along with sexuality and relationships, will be discussed.

Using words to define one's own life and describe components of one's personality is an empowering exercise for people who continue to be treated as invisible. It was ironic that the planners of a conference on self-determination would ignore their own mission and attempt to sanitize the message in the hope it would not offend some of the more conservative attendees. What occurred in the process was that the presenters, and the very attendees the seminar was designed to reach, were the ones who were deeply offended.

I believe the most powerful tool the gay community can use to effect change is also a personal one, which is to simply come out, tell our stories of growing up, and describe our feelings. The "closet" is a prison that has been effectively used against us, for anyone that considers his or her sexuality a source of shame (Bernstein, 1995). The resistance to come out is so powerful that many are unable to challenge what has typically been a lifelong assault. Because of the injustices I see and my experience every day as an openly gay man, I do not want anyone else who is gay, lesbian, bisexual, or transgender to be told they are anything less than unique and valued and cannot have a life filled with great potential.

### Future Goals

What I have most learned in this journey to provide a safe haven for GLBT persons with DD/MR is the power of the human spirit. Members who come to the RSG have endured some of the most inhumane conditions and difficult circumstances, yet their generosity and optimism shines at every meeting. Their insight into complex relationships is sophisticated beyond expectations. Their desire to build a sense of community is real as they respond to their own inner voices.

The RSG stands ready to serve as a model for human services professionals in other states and regions to create similar support groups for their clients. Already, the RSG has provided inspiration for other regions, Massachusetts and Minnesota, for example, as more human services staff recognizes diversity within the DD/MR community. The best course of action for the RSG is to simply continue doing what it has done successfully since September 1998—providing a safe and inviting environment for GLBT people with DD/MR.

During a recent conversation, a key administrator at one member's agency called to voice a concern that a frequent topic at RSG monthly meetings encouraged unrealistic expectations for this client. Since the client lives in an intensively supervised residential setting, it would be virtually impossible to allow any opportunities for intimacy or a close personal relationship.

"I can respect your position and will try to be more sensitive to your concerns," I replied, trying to remain cognizant that the comment came from an ally and not an adversary. I then added a caveat: "Having quality of life is more than just having a full belly and a warm place to sleep. Aren't we all looking for relationships and the opportunity to share our life with a partner?"

So what if a person lives under constant supervision? Is it not our obligation, as human services professionals, to ensure that people with DD/MR have the same opportunities to realize their dreams in life? Just as heterosexuals do not have a monopoly on sexuality, the potential for having a relationship is not limited to intellectual privilege—it is part of what makes us human. What the RSG has accomplished and will hopefully continue to illuminate is the understanding that people with DD/MR are entitled to a whole life experience, including discovering and enjoying their sexuality.

Chapter 2

# Professional Perspectives: Observations by Support Staff

"How do they know?" is a frequent response from people both within and without the health services profession when they first hear about the Rainbow Support Group. The question is at once innocent and insulting—an indictment of the patronizing regard society holds toward people with developmental disabilities.

How do people with developmental disabilities know they are gay? The same way individuals with developmental disabilities know they are heterosexual. It's as simple as they just do, by paying attention to what is going on inside of them (Marcus, 1993).

Members of the RSG discovered their sexuality the same way people without DD/MR discovered their sexuality. Their stories of coming out and acknowledging their feelings are no different than those told by other gay people. This awareness typically occurs over time, as the vignettes of life begin to reveal a sexual understanding different from society's dictates. People with intellectual disabilities know that they are gay the same way other gay people know—by being in touch with their feelings, through sexual experimentation, and, it is hoped, by participating in a shared community.

Members of the RSG speak of an early awareness of their sexual orientation, which is known as their coming-out experience. Most members, who are now between the ages of thirty and fifty, describe their coming-out experiences as having occurred between ten and fifteen years of age, compared to other gay people of the same age without DD/MR, who came out in their mid-to-late twenties.

## A Parent's Perspective

As an advocacy group for people with DD/MR, a Connecticut state agency supports several human rights committees in each of their five regions of the state. One committee member, who spoke on condition of anonymity, is an attorney and mother of a ten-year-old son with Fragile X syndrome and an IQ in the mid-fifties (a common form of mental retardation in males). She said that as a heterosexual married woman with strong religious views, she has not considered the sexuality of her son and is grateful the issue has not yet presented itself.

"It never occurred to me," she said and noted that since all of her son's relationships have so far been with staff, she hopes that one day he will develop friendships beyond staff and family. "I never thought of it, but chances are that he may end up in a single-sex home."

During the discussion, it was obvious this parent was considering for the first time the possibility of sexuality for her son.

"I would love for him to have a friend that was not me or my husband," she said. "And if he feels something special with that person, I think that would be wonderful, just to address the loneliness of people isolated, people just existing and not interacting."

She said that complicated issues such as sexuality are not given the attention they deserve and described a recent incident in which a client called a 900 number for the purpose of phone sex. The group home provider wanted it to stop, but did not base the decision on policy or financial reasons. Staff intervened because it made them uncomfortable to know their client was engaging in phone sex. They felt an obligation to thwart any sexual activity, regardless of the desire of the client.

"As far as I know, [the state agency] doesn't have a policy on this—sexuality. Issues are dealt with only when it becomes a problem," she said. "It's apparent to me that no one is giving the direct care staff policy information, either written or verbal."

She said staff could encounter a dilemma when attempting to provide opportunities for their clients that involve dating and sexuality. Arranging a date is an appropriate first step toward developing a close relationship, but in order for staff to feel protected in their job, they tend to be overly cautious and ignore common sense. Unfortunately, it is occupationally safer for staff to discourage such activities than it is to assist clients by providing opportunities for intimacy.

"Is it a denial of [the clients'] human rights to deny their sexuality?" she asked reflectively, then continued. "I think it is. We run into that within the [state agency] structure. People are concerned for their job, so they alarm the bedroom door or bed, because you don't want someone jumping into another person's bed."

She suggested that staff should assist clients in arranging dates.

"It's the same approach to social issues or being in a safe environment. They should have opportunities to socialize and staff should help facilitate dates," she said, but then offered a clarification. "I guess it is so individually based."

### View from the Couch

When the RSG came into existence, another group had been quietly providing support to GLBT people with developmental disabilities in New York City for two years. Simply called, "LGBT & Questioning Group for Individuals with DD," the group offered a three-tiered support structure, including psychotherapy, group therapy, and psychoeducation.

"The program director and I determined that many clients didn't have a place to go that was relevant to begin talking about issues of concern for this group," said Sean Flanigan, a drama therapist with a Manhattan-based human services agency.

Flanigan quickly built a group protocol with a twelve-week curriculum plan that included a statement of purpose, goals, how to run the group, and a list of topics for discussion.

"It came to the attention of the clinical staff at the [clinic] that gay, lesbian, bisexual clients needed a forum to experience themselves in a comprehensive manner, which took into consideration their sexual orientation, and to explore themselves on both the intrapsychic and interpersonal levels," said Flanigan, who has spent fifteen years in the human services profession. "Clinicians acknowledged the importance of connecting clients with other gay, lesbian, bisexual people, and community so that clients could begin the process of consolidating a [gay] identity."

Flanigan said it became quickly apparent that group members were grappling with the same issues other gay people have to overcome to find self-acceptance, as well as other concerns unique to their circumstances.

"The issues are that they're dealing with denial and terror and fear of their sexual orientation and not being able to find a partner," said Flanigan, who has maintained a close connection with the RSG and annually helps facilitate bringing the two groups together for a social function. "Don't most people want to share their life with someone? And our guys are no different. They are always saying, 'I want someone to share my life with.'"

However, Flanigan said he was unprepared for the self-conscious feelings many people with DD/MR harbor about their disability. "The main issue they are dealing with is the denial of their disability," he said. "There's a lot with that. I am impressed with the deep, deep, deep self-loathing they have toward their disability."

Flanigan said that when someone finds a partner, the individual is looking at a mirror, but what is reflected back for a person with DD/MR is the disability. "And it's intolerable," he said. "These men and women definitely know their place as the pariahs in the dominant culture. They are the object of ridicule and scorn."

Flanigan said the self-loathing message was brought to light recently when an intern assisting with the support group voiced an observation.

"The intern has observed in the meetings 'What about the gay issue?' It's not talked about," said Flanigan, who reported that even to a newcomer, the most pressing issue is the disability, not his or her sexual orientation.

"What touches them the most is they're severely disadvantaged, but they have such spirit to come to the meetings. It's what holds that hope and that there will be someone there in the future for them. It's what keeps them going," said Flanigan, who added that he finds it fascinating so many of the members know inherently that they are gay.

The RSG has presented each year at a large conference on DD/MR in New York City, and Flanigan was there to reconnect with the seven members who were presenting. During the opening comments, a brief profile of one of the members was read, which the member heard for the first time. By the second sentence, the member became inconsolably emotional, crying with deep heavy sobs. The moment was impressive.

"It was a very human experience. It is very painful just to live and they realize this is the one place I can come where I don't have to hide the mental illness, the disability, the gayness, and the common bonds are inherently therapeutic where we can just be with one another," said Flanigan.

"So in the meeting, when one is crying when he hears his profile and the other one is anxious, it means that they've fantasized about this moment. They've dreamt about having the opportunity to speak in front of a group," he said.

Flanigan said that for many members of the RSG and the group he facilitates, the underlying message is about being made visible for the first time in life.

"It's very powerful to tell your story and to have other people there to witness the story," said Flanigan. "They know that people came to hear them, and as retarded people, no one wants to hear what happens in their lives. The world tells us that we have to be beautiful, thin, and smart and retarded people don't fit that model. So when they have an opportunity to go to a conference where people have come specifically to hear what they have to say, that's a powerful and validating experience."

Frank Caparulo, a certified sexual therapist who works in Connecticut and New York, said that the profession has denied people with developmental disabilities access to sexual expression for too long. He said deprivation has only recently emerged as a human rights issue. "What the system wants is to keep people with mental retardation asexual," said Caparulo, a member of the American Association of Sex Educators, Counselors, and Therapists. "It's not about being liberal, it's about giving people the opportunity to experience their feelings and sexual needs."

Caparulo said that people with DD/MR are not permitted to participate in the rituals of dating and enjoy the pleasures and heartaches of intimacy, which is a learned behavior. He was critical of the profession for demonstrating a disregard for the pursuit of intimacy and romantic aspirations.

"There is a lack of respect for clients' sexuality—heterosexuality, homosexuality, any sexuality," said Caparulo, adding that the rules of sexuality are learned through experience, which is considered a taboo subject for people with DD/MR. "People say that I must be a good person to take care of the mentally retarded, but that doesn't go anymore. It's about recognizing that people with DD are people with normal sexual needs. There's nothing wrong with their sexual desires."

Caparulo said homophobia throughout the human services profession is a mirror of society's inability to accept homosexuality. The profession is just beginning to acknowledge that some people with

DD/MR are gay, lesbian, bisexual, and transgender as society has become more comfortable with the subject. Some agencies have devised a consent form that acknowledges sexual orientation—and sexuality in general—along with the repercussions of sexual behavior such as sexually transmitted diseases (STDs) or pregnancy and a new range of emotions. Caparulo also noted that individuals dealing with sexual orientation issues face additional hurdles which must be overcome before they can act on their desires.

"[People with DD/MR are] vulnerable to their own emotions, because they are not able to test their sexuality," he said. "When we are in high school, we learn that heterosexuality is the norm, but gay kids learn to distance themselves from their homosexual desires. We test this by having a girlfriend or a boyfriend. It's about sexual conquests, learning to make out and get some information. We go through the process to be successful in having sex. But gay kids are just too busy hiding out, and it takes all their energy."

Caparulo works three days a week at a Connecticut residential facility writing plans that sometimes involve sexual-enriching tools, such as adult novelty toys. He gave an example in which a resident in a group home had been observed inserting various household objects into his anus. Caparulo was called to evaluate whether the activity was self-injurious or pleasurable behavior. After determining the man enjoyed the activity, Caparulo offered a frank discussion on purchasing items that were intended for the activity. Equally important, he offered counseling to the staff, who may have had their first exposure to an explicit sexual discussion regarding a group home resident.

"People who work in institutions learn on the job, so they can make assumptions that aren't correct," he said. "They are given the label as caregiver and they take it literally, instead of supporting the people they serve, being sensitive, but also realistic about the potential of the individual."

The role of an advocate or caregiver is to model behavior and assist individuals with making good decisions. Caparulo felt that in more ideal circumstances, consumers would be allowed to enjoy recreational sex and explore their feelings. Other people without disabilities have those opportunities, but that as long as consumers live under the auspices of an agency, those choices cannot be presented.

"[The agencies] are either too conservative or hypocritical," said Caparulo, offering to explain why caregivers frequently take on the role of dictators, by squelching opportunities rather than helping the individuals discover their potential. "You don't just protect them all the time. You have to prepare them to deal with life's experiences. Part of it is listening to their heart, but also, you have to be realistic when reaching for the stars. We have to help them fulfill their personal dreams."

## *The Administrator*

The measure of an astute administrator is someone who creates a supportive environment to welcome positive change (Ladew, 1998). Agencies that provide support to people with DD/MR are conservative by their very nature because they are typically working with people unable to advocate on their own behalf. From the beginning of the RSG, when it was still just an idea, Joe Parente, vice president of the vocational division at a private agency in New Haven, was in a position to offer the full support of a leading agency behind the idea to establish a support group for GLBT people with DD/MR. The professional credibility offered by a private provider under the conservative DD/MR umbrella toward such a volatile topic as the RSG was an important first step.

"We'd like to offer support [for this project]," said Parente in April 1998 when asked if a flyer could go out under his agency's letterhead. The flyer announced the intention of several concerned individuals who wanted to form a statewide GLBT support group for DD/MR clients.

"I've been blessed with a close family, a spouse, and know how important that is to me," said Parente, reflecting four years later on his decision to offer administrative support . "You can see how the members want something similar—having companionships and relationships are so essential to life—but it can be so elusive."

Parente was aware of the many risks of lending support to the RSG and helping to initiate discussion on a controversal topic. He suggested steering initial contacts to top officials at the state agency and private, nonprofit agency executives so the message would be passed down from key policymakers.

"The group has to just focus on dealing with the core piece and not the political ramifications and then get as much information out as possible," said Parente, who is responsible for a large vocational day program for 150 adults with DD/MR. "We didn't take a step without letting the stakeholders know every step—the case managers, families, providers—even when it was not well received, but it was still respectfully received. [The state agency] was on board because they had time to process. That is particularly important when advocating something controversial."

Parente said that when several of his colleagues at other private providers heard about the activities of the group, they were stunned.

"They said things like, 'Holy cow, what are you doing?' But it went a lot smoother because of the process," he said.

Parente said that since people with DD/MR are considered asexual, their advocates must be prepared to acknowledge how sexuality impacts the daily lives of clients.

"You are dealing with people's personal value systems and response to sexuality," said Parente as he reflected on the relationships that have blossomed within the group. "The clients need additional supports because of their intellectual difficulties. You can see how they came together and over time [once they were more comfortable with discussing their sexuality], they were able to develop relationships."

Parente said watching members of the group and their desire to connect with other people like them left an indelible mark on his career.

"It is not insignificant that a group such as the RSG even exists," he said. "Before we can begin to answer whether [individuals are] competent to declare their sexual orientation, we have to acknowledge that they first have a sexuality. The right to healthy sexual expression is part of the human experience."

Even though he was involved only peripherally with regular meetings of the group, having a personal connection with its members assisted Parente in seeing them as whole human beings who had similar aspirations, regardless of their disability or sexual orientation.

"I've observed the challenges most people face blending their professional career and lifestyle and knowing how difficult that must be for someone with a disability who has been so excluded," he said. "They may have had difficulties developing relationships or confusion around their sexuality and knowing how those challenges are exponentially increased when brought together. You can imagine the frustration when the barriers multiply."

Many people with DD/MR live under close supervision not only in their vocational day programs but also within their residence. Constant supervision is not conducive to developing intimate relationships.

"Our lives are not so compartmentalized," said Parente, acknowledging the additional burden inherent in the lives of people with DD/MR. "Everyone wants fullness to . . . life and so this creeps into [other areas]. We have to set boundaries so the clients know to keep it in a private place, but at the same time knowing they don't have a private place."

Although many staff may be personally liberal and want to provide opportunities for their clients to develop relationships, Parente indicated they may feel compelled to be professionally conservative to avoid any situations in which policies are conflicted. As the activities of the RSG are publicized through the dissemination of literature and presentations at conferences, there is a higher level of acceptance among support staff throughout the state and an understanding that sexuality for people with DD/MR is a basic human right.

"That's where the work needs to continue with this particular issue," he said. "It points out the need to educate the community and staff within the residential programs. When things don't go well, the state agencies come down hard, because the risks are enormous."

### Support Staff

Advocates for people with disabilities are concerned with the well-being of the whole person, and sexuality is part of the human experience (Monat-Haller, 1992). Judy Goldberg, one of the founding staff members of the RSG, said she recognizes the importance of providing places where clients can express their feelings.

"As I've gotten involved, it's given me an education," said Goldberg, an employment services supervisor who works at a Connecticut vocational and residential agency for people with developmental disabilities and supports a client in the RSG.

"I've learned to recognize the diversity within my client base," said Goldberg. "Sexuality didn't come up in my area, because I'm in the vocational department, but I'm aware people are sexual. I'm comfortable with gay issues and I'm in a position to lend my support to provide a place for all clients."

As with other staff members who have helped make the RSG successful, Goldberg said part of the support she has provided has been through discussions with colleagues, clients, and their parents. "When I speak positively about the group and the topic, that allows others to think of the group positively as well," she said.

The RSG has been much more than a social outlet for members. Not only has it provided opportunities for members to discuss sexual activities in a more comfortable setting, it has also provided opportunities for staff to realize that sexuality issues can and do emerge in the workplace, such as when clients develop attraction toward one another. Through her involvement in the RSG, Goldberg has come to realize that sexuality issues can manifest in unproductive ways when they emerge in the workplace and are ignored.

"People with disabilities don't always know what is appropriate sexual contact and behaviors and they can put themselves in a potentially abusive situation," said Goldberg. "That's why the group is so helpful. It's teaching safety with vulnerable adults by helping them know who is a friend and how to define a friend, appropriate touching, safe sex, the Internet, and establishing trusting relationships."

Lynn Pearson (an alias), who recently joined the RSG's staff, is the vocational supervisor for one of the group's members. Pearson vividly recalled working with the member prior to his involvement in the group, when she said he was more vested in avoiding work. She observed a better work ethic once he began regularly attending the RSG.

"He's improved workwise," said Pearson, who has worked with the member for the past six years. "He always had a reputation for not doing his work, smoking, getting out of work, but not so much over the last year or two. We're not hearing the same kind of complaints or the frequency."

Pearson said that since she works in a vocational program, she is unable to facilitate social opportunities for clients. However, she is frequently aware of times when the lack of quality-of-life opportunities creeps into the work environment.

"People with disabilities are disrespected in their need and desire for relationships," she said. "Sexuality should not enter into the workplace, but the reality is that it does. I'm an out lesbian and working for people with developmental disabilities. It makes sense that I would be an advocate or a resource for gay people with developmental disabilities. This group brought it home for me."

Another founding staff member of the RSG who works in vocational services, Kate Campbell (alias), said that when sexuality issues are ignored or not adequately addressed, behavior problems inevitably surface.

"At a former employer, I said that we're starting a group for gay clients and they said, 'But we don't have any people like that,'" said Campbell, a senior employment specialist for a local vocational program. "I said, 'Oh yes, we do. We have the two guys that like to dress in women's clothing, and they're both gay, but not a couple.'"

"One tries to kiss guys on the van and everyone knows it," she said. She said that staff are reluctant to discard the women's clothing because it upsets the two men.

Campbell said some staff would quietly encourage clients to restrict their cross-dressing activities to the privacy of their rooms and redirect any displays of affection. The agency's response was to take no action in the hopes that by ignoring what was perceived as a problem, clients would find something else to occupy their attention.

"They said so long as he keeps it in his own room, that's okay," she said. "He would steal women's clothes from his family's home and steal from the company consignment shop. What I found strange was that the company always wanted to have innovative programming and be known in the local community for being innovative, but the agency in general is lacking in providing services in this area. They like to pretend the guys don't have a sexuality."

Campbell said that whenever GLBT sexuality issues surfaced, the administrative response was to steer the client into one of the other quality-of-life programs provided by the agency.

"Their response was, 'We have all kinds of other programs; we don't need this one,'" she said. "They have courses in daily living, hygiene, cooking, banking, job club, and recreation and dances, and I said, 'OK,' but they were all geared to heterosexuals."

She said that there was an implied policy at the agency to intervene whenever staff encountered same-sex activities, such as at company-sponsored dances.

"If two guys tried to dance together, it would be broken up, but if it was two girls, that would be okay, because it's socially acceptable for women to dance together in this country," she said. "I was concerned about gay profiling, which says that to be gay is wrong and should be discouraged."

The profession has been slow to change, but as the people being served learn the power of self-advocacy, Campbell said that the profession will be obliged to respond.

"I was always aware of the homosexuality in clients," she said. "In this field, you look at the whole person and see what you can do to make [his or her] life better."

### Rainbow Support Group Goes National

The Rainbow Support Group has taken its first step toward becoming a national organization. At least one other chapter has been meeting in Minnesota following a presentation in May 2001 at a statewide conference on disabilities in Bloomington, Minnesota.

During the first of two annual presentations, eighty people heard about the success of the New Haven-based group and the unprecedented issue of providing support and affirmation for people with DD/MR who identify themselves as gay, lesbian, bisexual, or transgender. Some of the conference attendees were interested in forming a group and were already aware of several potential members.

The first meeting of the RSG of Minnesota was held in September 2001. Just like the New Haven RSG, the group included gay men, lesbian women, and people who identified as bisexual and transgender. Since Minnesota is a large state, one member is driven from as far away as Duluth, which is 250 miles away, and another drives 100 miles from Mankato.

Without a centralized community center in the Twin Cities metropolitan area, the group has been meeting at gay coffeehouses, gay bookstores, bars, and at the various agencies where RSG staff are employed. An agenda has been established with various themes for discussion at the monthly meetings, including such topics and events as sexual health, coming out, gay pride, and movie nights.

"This is an idea whose time has come," said Marcus Linn, a program coordinator for a human services agency in St. Paul, Minnesota, and one of the founders of the Minnesota RSG. "When we as a profession help people, that means we need to help in every way and not just in areas that we're comfortable with. We want sanitized ideas of what life should look like. We don't have a right to deprive people [with developmental disabilities] of their sexuality."

Linn was critical of the human services profession and said it does the client a disservice when staff members are afraid to raise the issue of sexuality, whether based on their own discomfort with the subject or if they have prior knowledge that the topic is taboo with the client's family.

"We use guardians and parents as excuses not to try," said Linn, who has been with the same agency for eighteen years. "That's not to say that some people are not vulnerable, but we still need to try and allow them their own experiences. People have a God-given right to their sexuality and the right to form relationships."

One of the surprises for Linn after almost a year of meetings is the effect the RSG has had on staff connected with the group. He said that as the staff began supporting the members who participate in the monthly meetings, some of them came out professionally in the process as well.

The following is an anonymous promotional letter that was distributed at the statewide conference, May 29 through 31, 2002, Bloomington, Minnesota:

> As a staff person assisting my consumer, I find participating in the Rainbow Support Group very rewarding. I know from my own personal experiences that life can become so much richer when someone has the courage to follow what is in their heart. Finding the right partner can be an unfulfilled ache in a person's life. I am pleased and delighted to be part of this group; bringing a burning candle of hope to a few who had none before.
>
> I believe in quality of life with relationships being so much a part of that. Being different in our society has its own challenges. We have a few in this group that are different in more ways than one. They still have the same hopes and dreams that the rest of us do. I would hope that as a support staff person you would not let your own fears and bias get in the way of someone you serve having a fuller, richer life. Our group is a safe way for vulnerable adults to begin to share what is in their hearts with hope for the future. We provide friendship and support, with encouragement and lots of fun activities, too.

Linn, who is openly gay, said that he first became aware of the need for a support group during a company event three years ago, when a client approached him and came out to him in the discussion.

"At a company picnic, one of our clients came up to me and he had big earrings dangling from his ears," remembered Linn. "He said, 'Hi, I heard you were gay and I am too,' and we talked about his problems and how there were no programs."

Linn said that since the client was sexually active, he arranged to have him enroll in a six-week AIDS course called "Between Men." The course was taught by a local AIDS service organization where the client was able to hear positive messages about practicing safe sex, about sexual orientation, and about the risks associated with being sexually active.

"If we deny them access [to healthy sexual activities], then they are forced into pathological expression such as public sexual behavior or picking up drunks in a bar," he said. "We're much more adept at treating pathology and treating sexuality as pathology than helping people [with their desires]."

Once the group was formed and a core group of people began regularly meeting, Linn was candid in his observations about the group dynamics. He said that although he is pleased with the positive impact the group has had on its members, he is also guarded in his participation.

"You have to be really careful when working with people with disabilities," said Linn, who noted that some of the clients who come to the group are also just beginning to come out, which can be a process fraught with ambivalent feelings (Marcus, 1993). "I don't like to be alone with clients. I like to have other staff around, because people are willing to believe anything negative about queers. We've been conditioned as a society to believe that gay men are predators."

Linn said staff have attempted to steer the group away from meeting at gay bars and instead meet at coffeehouses or bookstores, but staff are also more interested in having members choose the location, and many members prefer to meet at gay bars. The one place members are adamant they do not want to meet is at one of the agencies where RSG staff are employed. Instead, members expect the meetings to assist them in accessing locations where other gay people congregate.

"They don't want to be associated with a center for people with disabilities," said Linn. "We have to provide access to the community, even if that means meeting in a gay bar. We even had one guy drop out because we were staying away from one of the primary gathering places of our community, which is the gay bars. We want this group to be consumer driven, and they are really vocal about where they want to meet."

Despite all of the reservations he had about helping to start a RSG chapter in Minnesota, Linn said he was amazed by the profound changes he has seen in members.

"I see changes happening monthly," said Linn. "[A lesbian member] has been writing articles about trying to have romance in her life and [a gay male member] finally was able to call a guy he is interested in and had an introductory conversation. We're encouraging people to do something we term *comfortable risk taking* every month."

Linn said he hopes the RSG will eventually become a national group with multiple chapters around the country. He envisions a speaker bureau and a national conference as a way to help more people with DD/MR, regardless of their sexual orientation, participate in self-advocacy and experience a more well-rounded life.

The following is an announcement of the newly formed RSG of Minnesota, written by Linn, that was distributed at the Minnesota 2002 annual conference:

> Following last year's conference, having attended the workshop/training re: GLBT support, a group of staff from several residential providers got together. We met to see how we could support gay, lesbian, bisexual, and transgender people who have developmental disabilities. Shortly thereafter, the first meeting of a GLBT support group for persons with DD met for the first time. This work group initiated and became the core group of the "Rainbow Support Group" of Minnesota.
>
> The RSG meets once a month on the last Wednesday of the month from 6 p.m. to 8 p.m. The location for each month's meeting, and the activity, is determined by the group. Many group members attend with staff that may participate in the group as well as provide transportation for the group member(s).
>
> The group has been meeting since September of last year, and has about nine members presently and we're growing larger every month. The members of the RSG value [one another] and provide mutual support and camaraderie. It is a rare opportunity for members to be open about themselves in a supportive environment, some for the first time. It is an eagerly anticipated

event every month. We love for new people to become involved, and for those of us who are service providers, this is an opportunity to support those people we serve to live fuller and richer lives.

As the group's facilitator, Linn said he has great empathy for RSG members who are trying to be true to their feelings and are at various stages in their coming-out process. His hope is for the group to remain active and be available for those who are sure to follow.

"We've all been there," said Linn, who said that even though he has always known he was gay, from as early as three years of age, there have been many times when he has felt isolated because of his sexuality. "Sometimes you can feel so alone. Hopefully, this group will help people with DD/MR see themselves in a new light."

Now more than a year after the group was founded, the most significant function of the group is that it exists and serves as an outlet for fellowship and a move toward self-actualization, Linn said.

"We need to reach out to people who aren't with us now, who are not out or who are not our friends," said Linn, who described the RSG as a synergistic support group that brings together disparate groups of people—men, women, people with DD/MR, staff, and community members. "Our strength lies in our diversity."

# SECTION II:
# THE MEMBERS

# Chapter 3

# Andrew

Scooby-Dooby Doo, where are you?
We got some work to do now.

There is a significance to 1969 that is not lost on Andy. For many gay people, it was during that infamous summer—June 1969 to be exact—that the modern gay movement began. More important to Andy, 1969 was the year he was born and the same year *Scooby-Doo,* his favorite cartoon debuted.

Andrew, who likes to be called Andy, is easily the member who has progressed the most. A founding member of the Rainbow Support Group who has faithfully attended every meeting and event, he was almost not allowed to participate in the group following its initial meeting. Andy's support staff felt he was too immature and unable to grasp the core premise of the group, which has always been to discuss what it means to be a person with a disability and also a member of the sexual minority community.

During that first meeting in September 1998, the facilitator went around the room giving everyone an opportunity to say something personal. Members took turns speaking and each was able to demonstrate that he or she had a self-awareness about his or her sexuality. They shared a sense of relief for finally being in a queer space—the New Haven Gay & Lesbian Community Center—where they were able to discuss their feelings. Mostly, they stated they felt alone and desired companionship. Companionship and loneliness are among the most popular themes at RSG meetings, and everyone that evening was able to articulate the reason they were there and what was going on inside of them.

Andy has difficulty speaking and being understood. He slides over his consonants, similar to the speech of the Great Dane cartoon detective, Scooby-Doo. When it was Andy's turn to speak, it was as if he was completely unaware of where he was and what others had just shared. He began talking about having a spaghetti dinner the previous night, when a staff person interrupted and reminded him of the topic. The moment caught the group off guard and, unfortunately, left the staff questioning whether he should continue meeting with the group.

Since he was a young boy, Andy has always known that he liked other males. He had his first sexual experience at age fifteen with a roommate at a now-closed state-sponsored residential school for children with developmental disabilities. The roommate was a streetwise boy three years his senior who liked to smoke cigarettes and easily engaged Andy in youthful exploratory sexual play. Andy said the participation was mutual, it occurred only a few times, and that he liked it. Although he did not identify the play as gay sex, he knew he could not tell the school staff at the time. So strong was the taboo for sex between people with developmental disabilities, and especially homosexual sex, that even now as an adult he still required assistance from his sister and legal guardian, Leslie, to retell the experiences. Andy actually seemed pleased when recalling those moments but had difficulty finding the right balance of words to express the pleasure he remembered and the shame he felt obliged to display for having participated in gay sexual play.

When Andy first came to the group, he identified as bisexual, since he had a platonic relationship with a woman he called his girlfriend. Shortly after joining the RSG, Andy began exploring how he identified and would at times refer to himself as gay.

"I told her that I go to group," said Andy in a matter-of-fact manner. "I told her my group is the Rainbow Support Group and it's for gay people. It's for men who like other men. And I like other men. I'm part of the Rainbow Support Group."

His girlfriend immediately broke off their relationship. The two have remained casual friends and Andy has devoted his attentions to developing relationships with other men, mostly within the group.

Andy's staff knew the RSG was appropriate for him since his actions explained what he could not express in words. Several years before, he had been caught engaging in sexual activity with another man in a public facility and had gotten himself in legal trouble. Many men, and not just those with developmental disabilities, who want to enjoy a shared sexual experience may feel the only outlets they have are opportunistic encounters in such clandestine locations as public rest rooms and parks (Blumenfeld, 1992). Unfortunately for Andy and others in similar situations, he was involved in a sting operation that resulted in a criminal record. He has since been sufficiently instructed to use a stall instead of a urinal when he goes into a men's room, even when he has only to urinate, since urinals are usually less private. Someone will check on him if he does not finish in an agreed-upon time.

Born into what seems like a typical baby-boomer family living in a medium-sized, working-class suburban community, Andy is the youngest of five children, whose ages range from thirty-three to fifty. He has two brothers and two sisters. His parents, who are both living, were married in 1951 and divorced in 1973. While he is emotionally close to his mother and guardian sister, Leslie, and maintains friendly relations with the rest of the family, there are darker moments in his family history.

Like many of those with developmental disabilities who attend the RSG, Andy has a history of sexual abuse. During the time he was sixteen to eighteen years old, his stepfather—his mother's second husband—molested him. Andy's sister, Leslie, said that in retrospect the family realized the stepfather was gay and coerced Andy into sexual encounters.

"My stepfather, sometimes he would come in my room and close the door," said Andy with a concerned look on his face.

Andy knows what was done to him was wrong, but he now feels that all gay sex is wrong, especially when combined with the incidents that got him into legal trouble. He grapples with the legacy of abuse and his desire to express his authentic sexuality in the present. To him, gay sex was what his stepfather did to him, and while he may or may not have enjoyed it, he clearly feels shame when reliving the experience.

Over the years of getting to know Andy, I have been profoundly impressed with his capacity for meeting people and maintaining friendships. Persistent and sociable, he is among the first to greet new members and, when given the opportunity, will incorporate a new friend into a regular routine of phone calls.

One of the ways I was convinced Andy had internalized the message of the RSG was his deliberate effort to maintain a scrapbook. He has become a strong advocate of the group and has assumed an unofficial role as the RSG's historian. He has saved every piece of literature and flyer relating to the group and has filled pages with photos that he coaxes from other members when they are passed around at meetings. He'll frequently rewrite RSG newsletters and newspaper clippings in longhand or on his home computer, which clearly gives him a greater sense of ownership in the group. By copying a newsletter or flyer, Andy further demonstrates his strong connection to the group.

Andy is quick to adopt current trends and is aware of fashions. He has a pierced ear and enjoys wearing contemporary jewelry. His favorite activity is to go to the movies. He is usually among the first to see newly released blockbusters and has a long list of favorite music groups, which are mostly boy bands such as the Monkees, NSYNC, and the Backstreet Boys.

To say Andy has a fascination with the cartoon *Scooby-Doo* is an understatement. When Andy is infatuated about something, he can go slightly overboard but in an innocent and fun way. He has a *Scooby-Doo* knapsack, *Scooby-Doo* notebooks and pens, and even boasts about wearing *Scooby-Doo* underwear. Although the infatuation may seem juvenile, it is not unlike any other infatuation people have with their hobbies. In the context of some other gay icons—Judy Garland, Barbie, Jackie Kennedy, even Tupperware—Andy's infatuation is understandable. He doesn't have to explain it, nor should he. Andy likes *Scooby-Doo* simply because he does, but like any other projection, we know that Andy sees himself in the friendly fun-loving character that never turns down snacks and always comes out the hero by the end of the show.

The cartoon centers around four teenaged detectives and a human-like Great Dane named Scooby-Doo, who has a scratchy voice and a comical laugh. The gang travels the country in a van solving dangerous mysteries. Scooby, as he is affectionately known, has many human qualities and is far from a perfect dog. He is something of a coward but manages to end each episode unscathed, praised for his coincidental genius, and, most important, the center of attention.

"I like Scooby-Doo, because he helps solve the mysteries," said Andy. "He's kind of a chicken, but he's really brave."

# Chapter 4

# Joe

"I've been out with so many of them, but it doesn't last long. We don't know who we want," said Joe, throwing his hands up in the air in a mock gesture of frustration.

"They have all considered each other," said Adrianne Prioleau, a residential counselor who has worked with Joe for five years. "It's a very small circle. If more members come, then they'll hook up with them, too. It's their only options."

The house where Joe lives is a tidy, sprawling split-level in one of the better neighborhoods of a medium-sized college town. With a well-maintained lawn, landscaping, and freshly painted siding, nothing seems to give away that this typical family homestead is now a group home for three men with developmental disabilities.

In many ways, Joe is an average guy pursuing the American dream. At first glance, he does not appear to be a person with a disability. Physically fit, always well dressed, and with a pleasant personality, Joe could easily pass as another considerate neighbor in a nice community. On one hand, he seems content with his station in life, and the fact that he has a disability does not seem to get in his way of enjoying himself, but Joe is resolute in his desire to have a boyfriend.

Joe is a quiet person and displays good manners. He is content hanging around his house and takes great pride in his room, which is comfortably decorated with furnishings he bought with his own money. Spacious and neat, his room is the master bedroom at the top of the stairs with a private bathroom. The room has an oak rolltop desk and an entertainment center with a stereo and a television where Joe can go for those moments he wants to have privacy. Over the dressers are posters of Ricky Martin and a Chippendale dancer.

"I like to shop, lots of shopping," said Joe, describing one of his favorite pastimes. "I like to wear clothes."

Hardworking and dedicated to his job as an attendant at a fast-food restaurant just down the street from the group home, thirty-seven-year-old Joe is able to make enough money to indulge his passion for shopping. Mostly, his shopping involves searching for trendy clothes, accessories, and music, but with his focus on finding a partner, his purchases have expanded to include small gifts of beaded bracelets and rainbow trinkets.

The phone has been a primary link for all of the RSG's members in their attempts to woo one another, and Joe is no different. On occasion, he has had his own phone and can easily spend hours talking with friends and potential mates, but the phone has also caused him financial difficulties. He currently does not have a phone and said it would be best for him to find a partner that lived nearby.

Joe said his residential staff helped him arrange a date with Ron, the youngest and newest member of the RSG, who lives forty miles away. Joe's staff drove him to pick up Ron, brought the two of them back to Joe's for dinner, and then took Ron home.

"I've never dated men before," said Joe, referring to his second date. "I've only dated men in the RSG. We picked up Ron and brought him here for dinner. He had a great time."

Joe said his first date with another man was a year earlier when he invited Andrew over for dinner for a similar evening. Joe's staff drove him to pick up Andrew, brought them back for dinner, and then drove Andrew back home.

"They have all considered each other," said Adrianne Prioleau, a residential counselor who has worked with Joe for five years. "It's a very small circle. If more members come, then they'll hook up with them, too. It's their only options."

Joe explained that part of his inability to develop a long-term relationship with one of the other members is they are all exploring and honing their relationship-building skills. The reason they alternate so quickly between one another is that they finally have a network of eligible men to practice dating and intimacy, even though their activities so far have all been rather innocent, since staff keep a close watch on any sexual content.

"I've been out with so many of them, but it doesn't last long. We don't know who we want," said Joe, throwing his hands up in the air in a mock gesture of frustration.

Prioleau felt the dating mélange perhaps added a diversion to an otherwise routine schedule. "This has turned into such a drama in their lives because there's not much else going on," said Prioleau. "I just want them at least have some of the same opportunities as anyone else."

Joe grew up in the same town where he now lives. His parents, both deceased, left his older sister as guardian and he has a close relationship with her. He rarely sees his two older brothers. Joe said he has had two long-term relationships with women—the first lasted eight years and the second five years—but they were both strictly platonic. The relationships served their purpose for companionship and conformity, but now that Joe is older and more confident in himself, he is able to more fully discover his personality with the assistance of understanding staff.

When Joe began acting on his same-sex desires, his staff recognized that he was more interested in connecting with men. Joe fully understands what it means to be gay and is candid in revealing that he has acted on his sexuality when opportunities were presented. Although he does not have a definitive coming-out story, Joe said that, in retrospect, he first learned about his homosexuality after he confided in a doctor as a young man.

"A doctor told me so," said Joe and then gave a confirming statement that demonstrated he understood his homosexuality. "I'm a guy that wants to be with another guy."

Joe said that he is given daily coaching to help him control his desires and to keep his emotions in check. He especially needs prompting as a reminder to demonstrate appropriate behavior toward other men in his work environment.

Joe said the qualities he wants in a partner are, at the very least, someone near his age who has a pleasant personality.

"My ideal person would have blue eyes, blond hair, smooth hair, no facial hair, no mustache, but they can have a disability, that's OK," said Joe. "I always wanted to be with attractive guys. It's kinda hard to find someone like that."

Currently, Joe has focused his attentions on Ron, who frequently calls Joe. The two have talked and are making plans to get together outside of the group.

"Ron, he's a nice guy. He's friendly, very polite. We talk about our first date, talk about getting together. I'd like to take him to a movie, but not a scary one. I'd like to take him out to dinner and a movie. I want him to be my boyfriend."

Joe said his ideal date would be to go to dinner and then see his favorite film, *The Waterboy*, starring Adam Sandler.

"Everyone always makes fun at him," said Joe, summarizing what he sees as the movie's core message. "His mother asked him where he's going. She's overprotective. He always goes to the football stadium. Everyone makes fun of him. When it's over, they show reruns [of the football game to the team]. In the end, he wins the game and becomes a hero."

# Chapter 5

# Ron

Wanted: Men Seeking Men
   Gay white male, brown hair, blue eyes, six foot, 170 pounds, looking for gay white male between 18-30 for friendship and possible relationship. Enjoy biking, walks by the beach, or quiet evenings at home. Serious replies only.
   Looking for a casual relationship. Likes: bike riding, romantic walks by the beach, and quiet nights at home. Looking for 18-35 and similar type of person. Smoker or nonsmoker—not an issue.

Having transportation is a rite of passage for many young men. A first bike or acquiring a driver's license or even learning a bus route offers cherished moments of liberation that encourage independence in a young person.

Ron never wanted a driver's license. He never wanted the financial responsibility that comes with operating a car—gas, maintenance, and insurance payments—but that has never squelched his desire to get outside, explore the region, and enjoy a sense of freedom.

Every member who comes to the Rainbow Support Group has a unique story to tell about how he or she came to participate in the group, but Ron's story is as complicated as it is engaging. His journey seems so atypical from what would be expected from a person with a disability.

Ron is a wonderfully polite person. He displays incredible patience, sensitivity, and good manners. At twenty-four years old, he has a contemporary sense of style, enjoys hearing the latest gossip, and tries to stay abreast of current events. He is tall at just over six feet, with a youthful look and thick wavy hair cropped short on the sides. He has big blue eyes, large white teeth, and an easy smile. He is also confident about his sexuality and deliberate in his search for a boyfriend.

Ron still lives at home with his understanding father and twenty-one-year-old younger brother, just a few blocks away from Andy. Ron's mother died at the age of thirty-seven from a reaction to medication when Ron was only seventeen. He doesn't like to talk about her death and said that losing her so young was especially traumatic.

"It was awful," he said. "I still cry about it; it gets me depressed."

Ron said he told his mother that he was gay a year before her death and he takes great comfort in making the decision to share his most private thoughts with her. He said that over time, it has become increasingly important to have had the opportunity to be honest with his mother.

"It was very difficult to do," he said. "It was at home in the living room. In the end, I just said it straight out. I told my mother as long as I can remember as a kid, I've been attracted to other men."

The revelation was an emotional moment for both mother and son.

"She had a typical response. She thought she did something wrong in raising me, but we talked a long time. The next day, I went on a bike ride with my father and told him," he said.

Ron has been diagnosed with attention deficit disorder and depression, and experiences great anxiety, which he says comes from having been bullied in school. School officials made arrangements to send him to a special-needs school after severe torment in ninth and tenth grades caused him to run away from home for two days. He finished his junior and senior years at a regional school two towns away.

"The kids said I talked slow and made fun of me," said Ron, referring to the first two years, which he said were exceptionally brutal. He was constantly on alert to protect himself. His life improved once he was in a new school and was able to make friends. He also became sexually aware and tried to fit in by dating girls.

"I felt a little attracted to women, but I was always attracted to guys. I was confused," he said, adding that he now knows that he likes guys his age, but also older men.

Ron has had two long-term relationships, both with older men. His first was with Tom (an alias), a professional man twice his age he met through a personal ad in the local alternative weekly newspaper. Ron described him as attractive, with a muscular medium build. Ron allowed the relationship to escalate more to satisfy his desire to have a boyfriend than his desire for this particular person.

During the two years they were romantically involved, Ron said he became increasingly unfulfilled in a relationship that was defined by Tom's whims and unscheduled changes. Their dates would be canceled at the last minute with no explanation or apology, and frequently Tom would simply not show up. Ron said Tom was a heavy drinker—usually vodka and orange juice—and would fall asleep before or during their date. When they finally did connect, it was usually for sex.

"Tom played mind games," said Ron, explaining his reason for ending the relationship. "He would stand me up or fall asleep when he was supposed to pick me up. Even now, he has done this again."

Ron said that although the affair ended, the two have remained cordial. Although they stay in touch with each other on the phone and have gotten together several times at a local diner, Ron still considers the relationship to be one sided. He resents feeling manipulated by his former partner but continues to call Tom during times when he needs a confidant.

At first glance, it is not apparent Ron has a disability. He is inquisitive and articulate with good language skills. An avid reader—Salinger's *Catcher in the Rye* is a favorite—he wants to become a special education teacher. He has great empathy for others and is generous with his time, possessions, and money. He does not drink alcohol, smoke cigarettes, or use drugs, and is aware of his sexual feelings. One of his many character strengths is his trusting nature, but that has also left him emotionally vulnerable in his constant search for a partner.

Ron has not always made the best choices in boyfriends. After breaking up with Tom, he immediately became involved with Brian (an alias), a receptionist who was six years older than Ron.

Ron met Brian through a telephone dating service and the two became fast friends. Their first date included a walk on the beach and a romantic kiss, but eventually their time together left Ron feeling empty. Ron said Brian refused to introduce him to his friends or family. Since both of them lived at home, their dates revolved around having sex in cars in parking lots or during times of the day when no one was home.

"Brian said that his parents don't like people with disabilities because they think they are not as smart as other people," said Ron. "He also never would introduce me to his friends because he said his friends made fun of disabled people."

"Do all gay men fool around?" Ron asked rhetorically. Brian once justified his infidelities by explaining that it was acceptable for gay men to play around.

Ron has a heightened sense of being victimized. He is concerned about the murder of Matthew Shepard, the Laramie, Wyoming, college student who was brutally killed for being gay, and says he does not watch television for fear of viewing broadcasts of antigay violence. "I'm scared [about the Matthew Shepard incident] because it makes me worry it could happen to me, because I'm gay," he said seriously concerned. "It could happen here. Gay people should be able to feel safe and show affection to others."

Twice he has gone to a local hospital to take an HIV test—both were negative—at the start of his new relationship with Brian and then again, after he discovered Brian was not monogamous.

Ron said he wants to better understand the gay community. His first lessons about sexuality came from high school health classes where the topics included lessons on heterosexuality only. He began to notice an attraction toward other boys at the age of fourteen and had his first homosexual experience at eighteen during a one-night stand.

Again, the two met after Ron placed the following personal ad in a local weekly newspaper:

Wanted: Men Seeking Men
Gay white male, brown hair, blue eyes, six foot, 170 pounds, looking for gay white male between 18-30 for friendship and possible relationship. Enjoy biking, walks by the beach, or quiet evenings at home. Serious replies only.

Looking for a casual relationship. Likes: bike riding, romantic walks by the beach, and quiet nights at home. Looking for 18-35 and similar type of person. Smoker or nonsmoker—not an issue.

The rendezvous occurred on a summer night where they met in a parking lot near Ron's house. "He was about my age. He answered the ad and I liked the way he spoke," said Ron, recalling that the other young man was cute and seemed nice. "We met in an empty parking lot and we had oral sex. I would have liked it to lead up to something.

I was wishing something could have developed out of it." Ron said that the experience was basically positive, but made him realize he preferred to have a relationship rather than quick encounters.

"I try not to have sex on the first date," said Ron, confident in the understanding that he does not want the yearning for a relationship to control his actions. "I want to become friends first and see what develops."

Ron said that even though he let Brian try to penetrate him, the experience was unsuccessful, since he was emotionally unprepared to fully share his body, but also because of the physical discomfort. Ron considers anal sex to be an expression of love reserved for a committed relationship. "I was afraid to have anal sex because of the promiscuity, and I want to save anal sex for my life partner," he said.

Ron came to the RSG at a low point in his life. Emotionally raw from the breakup with Brian and financially limited since his cavalier attitude toward employment had left him with a three-hour-a-week clerical job, he had little going on in his life and needed to feel grounded. His first RSG meeting was in February 2001, and it was electric.

Ron had been encouraged to join the RSG by several staff at his agency and was even invited to be a founding member. However, it took him two years before he felt comfortable enough to attend the group and was ready to begin meeting other people, including people with disabilities. Counting members and staff, there were eighteen people in the room.

A Valentine's Day dance for a youth group was just cleaning up when the session ended and RSG members were invited to enjoy an overabundance of pizza and snacks. The entire group stayed an extra forty-five minutes, milling around the buffet, socializing, exchanging phone numbers and e-mail addresses, and making plans to connect outside the group. The moment was memorable not just for its spontaneity but also for the sophistication the members displayed as they welcomed new members.

The evening presented an opportunity for members to visualize themselves in a new way, and clearly Ron was the catalyst. He was young and cute and appeared to be the least disabled of the group members. The greatest desire in a person with a disability, or at least for the members that attend the RSG, is to partner with a person that does not seem to be disabled. Many people with disabilities, and certainly the members of the RSG, consider their disability to be more of a liability than their sexuality and therefore do not want to be partnered with a person with an obvious disability. Suddenly, here was someone new that everyone wanted, the first person that passed for "normal," and since he was now a member of the group the others saw a potential partner in him.

# Chapter 6

# Andy Loves Joe Loves Ron Loves Andy Loves Ron Loves Joe Loves Andy

"I am attracted to [Andy]. I've started to care about him. I like the way he looks and his personality," said Ron, who then hesitated. "I don't want anyone to think that I'm a slut or dirty for going out with more than one person."

We both broke into a hearty laugh.

"I was thinking about going out on a real date with Andy, nothing big, to a movie, and also with Joe," he said.

Andy and Ron sat next to each other on the couch under the large picture window in the great room of the community center in August 2001. With a picturesque view of the sunset-drenched mountainside behind them, the facilitator, Maureen Thomas, went around the room inviting everyone to share something about their summers. Andy proclaimed that Ron and he were officially boyfriends. As he spoke, Ron sat next to him, attentive and nodding in agreement with a smile of satisfaction.

Romance is a universal language that has a normalizing effect for people with disabilities. Although the Rainbow Support Group is not a dating service, companionship and the search for a partner is the primary issue discussed during meetings.

The desire for intimate relationships is articulated by every member of the RSG, but for people with disabilities, courtship is a process filled with complications and hurdles. Dating can be difficult for non-disabled people, yet the process can become insurmountable for those who have to accommodate the additional demands of supervising staff who are dedicated to rules and routines. Too often, staff members maintain a posture of deliberate indifference toward tending to such desires, which can manifest in other unproductive behaviors.

People with disabilities are not encouraged to experiment with intimacy. "Person-centered planning" is jargon for dealing only with vocational and residential interests and benignly neglects dating and relationships. Sexuality, if discussed at all, is relegated to consultants who are specifically called when problems arise, such as someone acting inappropriately in public or displaying obsessive behaviors toward staff or nondisabled associates.

After five months, it became obvious that a three-way relationship had developed among Andy, Joe, and Ron. Each of the pairings had evolved through intricate connections that transcended the disabilities of the men. They are all evenly matched with similar interests and goals. All three are around the same age with similar intelligence. They all have their own sense of style, are conscious of contemporary fashions, and are all very focused on having a boyfriend. Most important, they all possess some unique qualities the others desire.

Although I served as a touchstone for the three men as they pursued their relationships, it was quickly apparent their dating behaviors were as sophisticated as any other personal relationship. The men had an awareness of the purpose for dating as they attempted to find partners, which is deftly presented next through a series of conversations and voice mail messages directed to me.

### Andy, May 21, telephone conversation

Andy called to say Ron approached him and kissed him on the face as a gesture of friendship and an intention to pursue a relationship.

"Ron kissed me, on the cheek," said Andy, who then stated his desire to have Ron as a boyfriend. "I like Ron, but he wants to date other people."

Regarding Andy's previous declaration of having Joe as a boyfriend, Andy said he has become increasingly frustrated over Joe's lack of interest.

"Joe doesn't return my phone calls," said Andy.

### Andy, May 22, telephone conversation

Andy called to say he was preparing to go to Ron's house for a supervised visit. Andy clearly wants a boyfriend and views Ron as a potential partner. He is constantly sharing that Ron wants to have sex with him and steals kisses from him.

The conversation got off to an exciting start with Andy saying that he was going to visit Ron's house and was expecting to have time alone with Ron. The two of them were planning to arrange an intimate rendezvous. However, when staff were contacted regarding the intention of the visit, their expectation was that this was simply a friendly one-hour visit since Andy was hounding staff about letting him spend time with his potential boyfriend.

Andy said that he was expecting to engage in sex with Ron and was looking forward to the opportunity.

"I'm fine with sex with Ron," said Andy.

I asked him whether he merely wanted to get together as friends with Ron or wanted to be with Ron like Pam and Dana, a lesbian couple in the group. Andy gave an emphatic response to the latter.

The names "Pam and Dana" have become code words in the group for partnership and sexual relationships and Andy clearly understood the two women were sexual partners. During the trip to New York City, he made kissing noises to explain why the two of them wanted to sit in seats behind the rest of the group on the train ride home, and he also made a hand gesture by holding his finger and thumb together in a circle and, with his other hand, poked a finger through the circle to symbolize intercourse.

"Do you just want to get together with Ron like Pam and Dana?" I asked.

"Uh-huh," he said in a slow and sly response that left no doubt of his intentions.

*June 6, Ron, personal visit*

For the first time, I became aware Ron was attracted to Andy more than just as a friend and I began to view the two as potential partners.

"Every day Andy calls me. He's cute and I'm attracted to him and his personality. I like to talk with him," said Ron. "He does things my ex-boyfriends never did. He pays attention to me and makes me feel good. He doesn't play mind games. It's just nice for a guy to pay attention to you."

Ron then mentioned he regularly speaks with Joe and sees potential with both men.

"Joe sent me a necklace last week," said Ron.

Ron said he and Joe write letters to each other every week, but he also talks with Andy every day.

One of Ron's former boyfriends has been a topic of interest during the phone conversations with Andy. Ron shared that Andy was interested in having a sexual experience with the former boyfriend and Ron at the same time.

"Andrew asked if [my former boyfriend], myself, and him can have a threesome," said Ron.

### Andy, June 11, before June meeting

Andy participated in a sporting event at a university in New Haven. Athletes from around the state stay in the dormitories for the weekend and Andy met someone from upstate and was excited to share the experience.

"I met someone from far away. He wouldn't give me his phone number," said Andy, who described an exchange he had with the other athlete in the fifth-floor showers.

"I went in first and he went in after me. I cleaned myself. He rubbed my leg under the shower stall. Then he touched my penis with his hand. Then he wanted me to go into the bathroom," said Andy, taking great care to describe the sequence of events.

I asked him whether he wanted to participate in the activity or had it imposed on him. "Oh yes, I did," he said, with a Cheshire cat grin and nodding his head. "I had my Scooby-Doo underwear. He wanted me to do sex and I said yes."

Having shared the story, Andy said he saw Joe at the pool.

"Joe wants to get back together," said Andy, without breaking his concentration on the events of the past weekend. "He has a nipple ring."

### Ron, July 23, telephone conversation

Ron called to say that he has been thinking about Andy and realizes he is attracted to him. He met Andy at the February meeting six months earlier and is aware of the strong feelings he has for the man who lives just a few blocks away and is supported by the same agency.

"I want to start a relationship with Andy," said Ron. "Hopefully I found someone who is faithful and doesn't play any mind games. I want someone that I can spend my life with."

Ron has been having telephone conversations with both Andy and Joe. When he told Joe about his former boyfriend, he gave the boyfriend's phone number to Joe and the two of them have been speaking on the telephone.

"[The boyfriend] was a lousy boyfriend but a good friend," said Ron, who then said he regretted giving out the telephone number and hoped it did not get anyone in trouble. He also said that Joe's counselor, Adrianne Prioleau, was unaware the two were phone buddies.

"I've had feelings for Andy for quite some time that were more than friends. I told him that I had feelings for him, but was afraid of them. After thinking about it, I decided I want to have a relationship. I've been lonely for a very long time and it's nice to have someone special," he said.

*Andy, July 23, telephone conversation*

Andy called, excited to share his news for the day. He has been spending more time with Ron and the two of them are becoming close friends.

"Ron just came over. We kissed in the backyard. It was a big kiss. He told me, 'I love you'," said Andy, who then described what he has been conditioned to do with any request out of the ordinary. "I'm going to talk [to my residential director] so we can be alone."

*Ron, July 29, message*

Ron called and left a message that he had spoken with Andy's staff about setting up a meeting so that he and Andy could arrange opportunities for private times.

*Ron, August 14, message*

Ron left a message that he was upset with Andy's staff and was increasingly frustrated about the difficulties he has getting through to Andy.

Ron said Andy's staff were often rude to him. He shared his frustration with Andy, but instead of sympathizing with Ron, Andy got upset with him and threatened to hang up. Ron then hung up on Andy.

*Ron and Andy, August 15, 16, 17, telephone conversations*

Over a three-day period, Ron and Andy had a divisive argument that threatened their friendship. This argument serves as an example of how important it is for staff to allow individuals to make their own friends. In a series of telephone calls to my office, each sought to use me as an intermediary to explain his actions toward the other. The volley was exasperating but offered direct access to each of them, to hear their concerns and witness an important passage for people who were never given permission to explore intimate relationships. I found myself trying to respect their confidences but also felt compelled to be a diplomat and help them quickly return to being good friends.

Andy was the first to call and was extremely upset and defensive. In a mixture of emotions, he displayed anger at Ron, frustration over their recent exchange, and fear that somehow there would be retribution from his residential staff or me for having an argument.

"Ron hung up on me," were the first words spoken by Andy without giving his usual greeting.

Ron called a few minutes later and offered his version of what happened. Ron said he tried to call Andy for a friendly conversation and no one answered the telephone. He said it rang for a long time and when someone picked up the telephone, that person immediately hung up. He said he then called the staff telephone, which is restricted to official business.

"I called Andy's house on the staff line and the staff person on duty was rude to me," explained Ron, who was equally upset and eager to volunteer the exchange that just occurred a few minutes earlier.

"Andy got mad at me because I was upset with his staff person. He started yelling at me. I hung up on Andy because Andy said he was going to hang up on me," said Ron.

The next day both Ron and Andy called and I suggested they talk, apologize to each other, and lay down some ground rules about how best to visit and talk on the phone. My suggestions included setting another time for speaking if one of them was too busy to talk. I also implored them not to hang up on each other in a rage and not to yell at each other. Their telephone calls should be respectful and fun, otherwise, they should not call in the first place.

On August 17, they both called again. Ron called in the morning and said he was back with Andy and hoped to have a meeting soon with Andy's residential staff manager to determine if they can have opportunities to spend private time together.

Andy called in the afternoon and said they had made up, went outside behind the tree (which shields them from the view of staff), and kissed. Andy said they talked about sharing a room together if the group goes to Provincetown together next summer on vacation.

*Andy, August 15, message*

"Me and Ron had a fight last night on the phone. Please call me back."

*Andy, August 15, message*

"[It's] Andy. I need to talk about something about Ron. He's yelling at me again. I don't want him, not a boyfriend in my life. Please call me back soon."

*Ron, August 16, message*

"Hi, John. I called to say I've straightened everything out with Andrew. We talked things over and said to each other that we weren't going to hang up on each other anymore. I promised him I wasn't going to call on the staff phone and we're going to set up a time when we can both speak to each other. Andrew and I worked everything out. Bye."

*Ron, August 21, message*

"Hi, John. It's Ron. It's nine o'clock Tuesday evening. Andy just called me and broke up with me. He said that he wants to be with some other guy and he told me he just wanted to be friends with me and I tried to ask him why. I mean, why he wasn't happy with me, and he got mad and he hung up on me. So, you know, I'm just a little upset and need somebody to talk to. You know, I tried to ask him in a nice way why he wasn't happy with me and he got mad and hung up on me. So it doesn't look like Andrew and I are together anymore. I'll try you again tomorrow at the office. I'll talk to you soon. Bye."

### Ron, August 22, telephone conversation

Ron called in an emotional state, crying that he was just dumped by Andy. "Andy called me last night and said he was breaking up with me," said Ron in a depressed, monotone voice. "I seem to keep getting involved with guys who keep leaving me for someone else."

Ron said Andy broke up with him because Andy wanted to be free to see other people. Ron said that one of Andy's staff had suggested that Andy may be interested in one of his friends and was planning to fix him up on a blind date. Therefore, Andy told Ron he was unavailable.

"When I asked him why he was breaking up with me, he hung up on me," said Ron. "I was made fun of since junior high and I have a lot of anger. I don't understand why people are so mean to others, why they hurt their feelings. Because of that, I'm very insecure."

Once again, I shared how important it is to exhibit good phone manners and be respectful of each other's feelings. I reminded Ron how frustrating it can be when someone gets hung up on, such as what he did the other day to Andy when they had the argument. Although I did not condone the action, I thought Andy had hung up on him as retribution for the other day.

### Andy, August 22, telephone conversation

Andy called with a deliberate and defiant tone in his voice. He called to report the events of yesterday's encounter with Ron.

"We had a fight yesterday. He's too much for me, his attitude," said Andy. "Ron is going to Rainbow Support Group and we'll be friends and that's it."

The apparent cause of the argument centered on Andy's staff member suggesting that Andy should not settle for one person yet. Andy said he was upset because Ron was trying to force himself on Andy and engage him in sexual activity. Andy implied this was wrong.

"He wanted to jump my body," said Andy. "He wanted to have sex with me."

I reminded Andy it was fine if he did not want to be boyfriends with Ron and that he did not have to have sex with him. It was also OK if he did not want to be friends with Ron, but the argument they were having was precisely the reason they should take things slowly. Intimate relationships grow from two people being friends first and if Andy and Ron will ever be boyfriends, they must first be good friends. I told Andy to continue to enjoy Ron as a friend and see him at the monthly group meetings and stop worrying about finding a boy-friend. I told to him I know it sounds old fashioned, but if he truly wants a boyfriend, it will happen someday when he is ready. For now, he should just relax about looking for a boyfriend and concentrate on the group and meeting new friends.

*Ron, August 24, message*

"Hi, John. I was just wondering if you've spoken with Andrew or if he gave you an explanation about why he hung up on me. I don't mean to put you in the middle of it. I'm sorry but I was just wondering."

*Ron, October 2, message*

"Hi, John. It's Ron. I'm sorry to be bothering you so much. I called [my agency] to find out when Andrew's next social club thing is so I can join them in that, if I'm not working, and also I'm going to call the Greyhound bus company tomorrow to find out if they can send a schedule in the mail and I might try to see if I could go up to see Joe or else if I see Adrianne at the group I might talk to her and see if I can make an arrangement with her to visit Joe and I also wanted to thank you for all the advice that you've given me and all the help you've given me. I'm looking forward to seeing you at the Rainbow Support Group on October 8, and if you'd like to give me a call when you get a chance, you can. Thank you very much. Bye."

*Ron, October 16, message*

"Hi, John. It's Ron. I have a couple of things I want to talk with you about. I just talked to a friend of mine who I was dating a few years ago and his parents don't want me calling there any more because they're very religious and they're the type of people who think that homosexuality is a sin and [he] told me his parents don't want me calling there anymore because I'm gay, you know. I just said to [him], 'Fine, you know, I won't call you anymore,' and he said he's going to call me and now all of a sudden he's saying he just wants to be friends. And the past few months he's been trying to get me to go out with him and now he just wants to be friends.

Anyway, I'm sorry to be leaving such a long message, but could you give me a call back when you get a chance? Bye."

### Ron, October 24, message

"Hi, John. It's Ron. It's twelve o'clock on Wednesday afternoon. I'm still in [town] and just about to catch the bus, so I don't know if I'll be home by one o'clock so I'm just going to tell you how the rest of the meeting went. It went pretty well and Andrew and I are just going to take things really slowly now and then when we both feel like we want to be intimate, we're going to have you and [Andrew's staff person] and Andrew's [guardian] at a meeting and discuss things, but the meeting went really well and [Andrew's staff person] apologized and he shook my hand and everything's okay now. Bye."

### Ron, October 24, telephone conversation

Ron called to say he had a meeting yesterday with Andy's residential director to share the frustration he experiences when he calls for Andy. The meeting included the director, a male direct care staff that he has had difficulty with, and himself. The meeting lasted fifteen minutes.

"I started to tell [Andrew's residential director] how I felt. She asked if everything was resolved with [Andrew's staff person]," said Ron, who then explained that [the staff person] told him Andy was not home the other day when actually Andy was. Ron said the deception was deliberate.

"I was a little nervous confronting [Andrew's staff person], but he never got upset," said Ron. "If Andy and I eventually do have a relationship, I don't want any problems with staff."

Ron said the outcome of the meeting was positive. The staff person apologized and Ron accepted it.

"[He] apologized and said he was sorry if he came across as rude. [Andrew's residential director] said that sometimes the staff can be short without meaning to be. I accepted the apology and we shook hands." The meeting also included a brief discussion about intimacy and dating.

"[Andrew's residential director] said I could see Andy when I want and she will assign staff to take us to a movie," said Ron, who added he and Andrew will have to arrange a motel visit if they want to be alone.

"There is no sex in the house," he said. "I wanted to go out with Andy and get to know him better. I know what we did out back was wrong and we won't do it again, but we didn't have anywhere else to go."

*Ron, October 25, message*

"Hi, John. It's Ron. It's ten o'clock Thursday morning. I was just wondering if you had a chance to talk with [Andrew's residential director]. If you got in touch with her and what was said, can you get back with me when you get a chance? Thank you very much again for giving me the advice and for helping me. You've been a really big help and I appreciate that. Thank you very much."

*Ron, October 29, message*

"Hi, John, it's Ron. It's eleven o'clock on Monday morning. I hope you had a nice weekend. I don't mean to keep bothering you. I'm sorry about that, but I was just wondering if you could let me know when you talk to [Andrew's residential director] and let me know what she said. The Halloween party was great on Friday. Andrew and I had a really nice time and it was really enjoyable. Anyway, I hope you had a nice weekend. I'll talk to you soon. Looking forward to seeing you at the next support group meeting. Can you call me when you get a chance? Thanks. Bye."

*Ron, October 29, message*

"Hi, John. I'm sorry to bother you. I was just wondering if you knew the phone number—the staff phone number for Joe's group home. Joe left a message on my machine and we kind of keep missing each other every time he calls me. I'm always out and I was just wondering if you knew the staff number at Joe's group home. Could you get to me when you get a chance? Thank you very much. Bye."

*Ron, October 30, telephone conversation*

Ron called to ask for Joe's new telephone number, which Joe has not shared with Ron. Joe has been calling Ron to arrange a date.

"Joe's been leaving messages asking me to call him back. Joe and I are supposed to go out on a date for dinner and a movie and Adrianne said that we would have to arrange it," he said.

I asked Ron how he and Andy were doing. He expressed frustration with Andy, who insisted on pursuing their relationship, yet remained aloof and talked about other potential partners. Ron was upset that Andy had befriended another athlete at the sporting event in New Haven and had engaged in a tryst in the showers.

"I'm not saying Andy is dumb, but do you think Andy understands the concept of relationships?" he asked. "One time he talks about being with me and then another time he talks about getting together with the person that touched him last year at that sporting event. I would never say that he's dumb about anyone because I wouldn't want anyone to say that about me."

I told Ron I thought he was discussing fidelity. Andy has never had the opportunity to have a boyfriend or a long-term partner. The only sexual experiences Andy had were casual, clandestine encounters seized during the few moments he was out of view of diligent staff. I felt what Ron described was not Andy's inability to understand commitment but rather, Andy's first exposure to someone interested in pursuing a long-term relationship. In other words, Andy had no reference point.

"I am attracted to [Andy]. I've started to care about him. I like the way he looks and his personality," said Ron, who then hesitated. "I don't want anyone to think that I'm a slut or dirty for going out with more than one person."

We both broke into a hearty laugh.

"I was thinking about going out on a real date with Andy, nothing big, to a movie, and also with Joe," he said.

I told Ron I did not think of him as a promiscuous person and explained that what he had described was a ritual of dating. Ron enjoyed the fact there were two men he found attractive and wanted to know if it was acceptable to pursue them both at the same time.

"That is why they call it dating," I said. "Dating is what people do to explore the possibility of a relationship, but it would be another story to get involved sexually with both of them."

*Andy, November 2, telephone conversation*

Andy called to say he had dyed his hair blond, like one of the singers in the Backstreet Boys.

"Ron likes it," said Andy. "He kissed me on the front porch. We're going to try to go on a date. We don't have any money."

Andy said he likes Ron and wants to spend time with him.

"We're going to take it slow at first, just like you said," he said.

*Andy, November 5, telephone conversation*

Andy first gave me a five-minute recap of his activities over the weekend. He went to the movies with his housemate and staff, continued to enjoy his dyed blond hair, and said he does not always have time to see Ron. He said Ron stops by on the way home from work. Since Andy has house duties, he is not always free to spend time with Ron.

I cautioned him that if he wants Ron in his life more as a boyfriend than a friend, he would have to plan and arrange a time and place where the two can get together. Otherwise, Ron may become disinterested in pursuing a relationship.

Andy then wanted to talk about last night and became emotional talking about how he does not have privacy in his own home. He feels tremendous frustration over house rules that require all bedroom doors to remain open. He can never enjoy a sense of complete privacy in his own room.

"I was thinking about men," said Andy, his voice cracking with emotion. "I want to be with a man in my room. I want to be with Ron, but I can't close the door."

We talked about arranging a meeting with his staff to seek a compromise on privacy. Although he has been instructed about inappropriate public behavior regarding masturbation and public sex, he is not permitted a private place where he can entertain guests and enjoy a private and intimate relationship.

*Ron, November 8, telephone conversation*

"I went on a date with Joe yesterday," said Ron immediately after we exchanged greetings. He was excited to tell me his news. "Adrianne picked me up at three o'clock."

Joe's counselor, Adrianne Prioleau, drove forty miles to pick up Ron, and bring him back to Joe's house. Prioleau cooked them dinner and drove Ron home after dinner.

"She made dinner—manicotti, salad, and pumpkin pie for dessert with whip cream topping. I got back a little after eight. Not many staff would do that. I was thinking of sending her a thank-you note."

Ron said that while Adrianne was preparing dinner, he and Joe watched a movie and talked.

"We watched the movie *Grease*," he said. "It's a pretty good movie. I saw it before and forgot how good it was."

In between the moments alone, Ron said that the conversation focused on relationships. Joe inquired about Ron's past relationships.

"He was talking about relationships. I kind of warned him about my past. He hopes someday I can be his boyfriend," said Ron. "He gets depressed because he's never had a boyfriend."

Ron's response to Joe was the same message RSG members have heard me repeat time and again.

"I said it's best if we take it slowly and see if things work out," said Ron. "He has the qualities of what I want—fidelity and honesty."

When it came time to say goodbye in Ron's driveway, Ron said the moment was unexpected and romantic. Joe lives in a group home and his two housemates had to come along for the ride. They were sitting in the van with Prioleau.

"Joe walked me to the door. I thought it was nice of him to walk with me," said Ron. "He hugged me goodbye. I thought that the others were watching us, but I didn't feel uncomfortable. He gave me a scented silk rose at the door. I though it was a nice gesture. That's my idea of how a date should be—dinner, a movie, and talking."

Ron said that he wanted to go on another date with Joe, which would hopefully be out to dinner, or somewhere in public. He was concerned, however, that staff would have to accompany them since Joe does not read or tell time.

Ron seemed more excited about the attention received from Joe and his staff than Joe as a person. He finds Andy more attractive than Joe, but is put off by Andy's indifference and inexperience.

"I don't want to sound shallow. I hope you don't think I'm shallow, but I find Andy more physically attractive," said Ron. "I like the way he combs his hair; he's cute. He looks cute with glasses on. There's more bulk to Andy—Joe is more slender."

Ron said he does not expect to share with Andy his date with Joe. "I don't know if I'm going to tell Andy," he said. "Andy hurt my feelings when he kept talking about other men. I would never do that to anyone else."

## *Ron, November 13, message*

"Hi, John. It's Tuesday morning. I wanted to talk with you and ask you if maybe I should call [Andrew's residential director], too, and try to set up a meeting with her. I'll wait to hear from you to see what you think about it before I call her."

## *Ron, November 13, telephone conversation*

A meeting is supposed to occur with Andy's staff, family members, and Maureen Thomas, the RSG facilitator, to discuss the potential for Andy to have more privacy, specifically with Ron. The meeting has been a discussion item for the last month as various parties played telephone tag.

"I've been doing a lot of thinking lately and would like to have that meeting," said Ron. "Every time I see Andy, there's a strong attraction to him and I'd like to have a meeting. I think he's pretty hot. I'm going to order him a Scooby-Doo sticker set."

Ron described the reasons why he enjoys Andy. Ron is most attracted to Andy's physical appearance and friendly nature, since Andy welcomes every new person who comes to the group. He said his one caveat about Andy is Andy's interest in meeting other men for the purpose of sexual experiences.

"He's a nice guy, but maybe I could show him, teach him about monogamy," said Ron. "We should be able to have our privacy. I don't like to sneak around."

*Ron, November 14, personal visit*

Ron made a personal visit. He was selling Avon catalog products to earn extra money for the holidays and used the opportunity to discuss recent events with Andy.

"I called Andy last night. He was in the middle of a video game and said he couldn't talk long. He said he's sorry about asking about going into the bathroom to do stuff. He didn't need to apologize, just that it wasn't the time or place to do that," said Ron. "We didn't do anything but kiss on the lips, just a quick kiss. I really enjoyed kissing him and he really enjoyed it too."

Ron described the dilemma he was experiencing, which was his attraction to two men at the same time and how best to pursue relationships. "I'd like to continue being a friend to Joe and see him as a friend, but I want to continue to pursue being more than friends with Andy," he said. "Andy's never really had a serious boyfriend and I'd like to help him understand that better."

*Ron, November 14, message*

"Hi, John. It's Ron. Andrew called me today and I also spoke with [Andrew's residential director] and Andy told me he's not ready for a committed relationship yet and Andy just wants to be my friend for now and nothing more than that. And I told both of them that that's okay and that I'd still like to be Andy's friend, and so Andy and I are just going to be friends. I mean, I'm a little bit disappointed and a little bit upset, but you know I'll be all right. I was really hoping that Andy and I could have a relationship and so I guess we can forget about that meeting now. We don't need to have that meeting anymore and [Andrew's residential director] said she was going to call you back. I just spoke to her and I gave her your phone number at the office. If you want to give me a call back when you get a chance, you can. Thank you very much, John. Bye."

*[Andrew's residential director], November 14, message*

"Hi, John. How are you? This is [Andrew's residential director]. I got your message via Ron. I haven't really listened to my voice mail, because I haven't really been in the office, but he said to me, because he was here when he was talking with Andrew, that you had tried to call me earlier and I also got a message from [the receptionist] that you've been trying to call me. But I have not received any voice mails from you that you've been trying to reach me, so I was surprised to hear that. However, I just had a conversation with Andrew and I had a conversation with [Andrew's guardian] and she's going to give you a buzz at some point when she gets a chance, but as far as this meeting for—that Ron was talking about, I'll wait until you hear from [Andrew's guardian] and then you can decide if we need to have a meeting in regards to privacy. The guys have about as much privacy as they can have in a group home, and one thing that concerns me is that they want to get intimate-intimate, which, from my understanding—the last time I spoke to Ron—he wasn't ready for that and I don't feel that Andrew is ready based on what he's telling me today. He said actually that, that's not something he wants to do, so we need to talk for sure so that, because I don't want him being stressed out because he can't decide what to do about a relationship. So, I'll give you an attempt again to touch base and then see what we can do. OK? Bye."

*[Andrew's guardian], November 14, telephone conversation*

After sharing some of the phone and message exchanges between Andy, Ron, and me, I suggested to Andy's guardian that she call a meeting regarding the privacy issue for Andy. While Andy's guardian knew Andy and Ron were friends, she was unaware of the significant involvement between the two. She said Andy has not spoken to her about his relationship with Ron and has not brought the subject up when he comes to her house every other weekend. However, she has consistently told Andy she will support his desires and decisions within reason.

"He has not shared anything with me, but he's always fearful that he's somehow going to disappoint me in some way. He's always looking for approval," she said.

She questioned Andy's readiness for a relationship and whether he was ready to live in his own apartment in a less restrictive living arrangement. "I don't know if Andy's ready for intimacy and if he knows what that involves," she said.

I told her Andy understood about safe sex, condoms, kissing, touching, and mutual masturbation. Andy had shared with me privately on several occasions, including a moment during the RSG meeting three days earlier, that he wanted to pick up more free condoms at the community center. I told Andy's guardian about Andy's conversation with me, during which he had become emotional about touching himself in his bed while thinking about Ron and told me how frustrated he was that he can never close the door to his own room to entertain a guest.

"I'll have to speak with him before I'll agree to a meeting. Andy has to tell me what's going on first. I'll plant the idea in his head first to let him know that he can tell me what's going on and then when he knows he can tell me, he usually comes around in twenty minutes," she said. Andy's guardian revealed she knew something was wrong during her last visit with Andy, but he never said what it was and she thought he was mad about something else.

*Ron, November 15, message*

"Hi, John. It's Ron. Andy called me yesterday and told me he's not really ready for a committed relationship yet. He just wants to be friends with me and then [Andrew's residential director] came on the phone 'cause I didn't really understand a lot of what Andy was saying so [Andrew's residential director] kind of clarified everything for me. So I don't think we're going to need to have that meeting. Andy and I talked also today on the phone. He said he'd still like to be friends with me, but that's it. So I don't think we need to have that meeting after all. I'm a little bit disappointed because I really like Andy and I was really hoping I could have a relationship with him, but I guess I'll just look for somebody else or try to find somebody else, and maybe I'll try to go on another date with Joe and see how that goes. If you want to, give me a call when you get a chance. Thank you very much. I'm sorry to bother you again. Bye."

*Maureen Thomas, RSG facilitator, November 19,*
*telephone conversation*

The ability of members to have access to privacy is a common subject at RSG meetings. Mostly, the topic surfaces in the form of reminders from staff present at the meetings that if members become involved in an intimate moment with someone, it must be done in an appropriate place.

Andy and Ron had engaged in several intimate moments in Andy's backyard where they kissed and touched one another. Although their activities were shielded from view of the house staff, they were in full view of an adjacent apartment building.

After the incidents were discussed within the group, Maureen Thomas, psychotherapist and facilitator of the RSG, said she was interested in participating in a meeting with Andy's support staff and guardian. I told her about the recent conversation I had with Andy's guardian.

Thomas's response was blunt.

"Maybe [Andy] is immature, but the problem is that he's sexually active," she said, acknowledging that Andy is candid about his sexual activities and desires and knows the RSG group is an appropriate place for such a discussion. "But you can't fight for someone who won't fight for themself."

### *Andy, November 19, telephone conversation*

Andy called to share the conversations he had over the weekend that brought a sense of closure to his courtship with Ron.

"We're not going to be boyfriends no more," said Andy.

I asked him why not.

"[My guardian] said, 'Don't do it no more with Ron'," he said indicating that he and his guardian spoke over the weekend about his relationship with Ron and their activities in the backyard.

I asked Andy how he felt about the decision.

"A little sad by it, but Ron has [another friend]," said Andy in an especially brief conversation that we both knew signaled the end of his courtship with Ron.

### *Postscript*

Following the ending of the courtship between Ron and Andy, a brief relationship sprouted between Ron and Joe. The two new partners began regularly writing letters and calling each other during the winter months.

Ron told Joe he enjoyed their time together but did not consider Joe a romantic partner. The two had a heated conversation one early spring morning and Ron called to talk about their telephone call.

"Joe called me this morning and said that he is upset that I don't feel the same way as he does," said Ron emphatically. "I've always told Joe I'd like to be his friend. You know, within a week of meeting him, he started telling me that he loves me. I don't think that someone can know if they love that person after only a week."

Ron said Joe had colored his hair with streaks of blond and had called to arrange a date to show off the new look.

"He colored his hair and then called me," said Ron. "He must have thought it had something to do with his looks. I look for their personality. Joe is a nice guy, but I don't feel anything romantic with him."

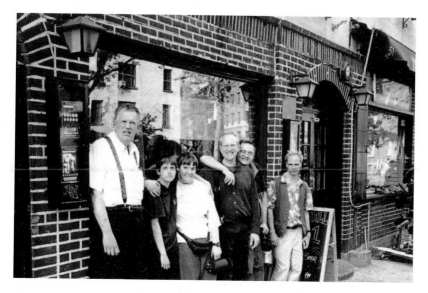

From left to right, Allen, Pam, Dana, John Allen, Andy, and Steven pose in front of the Stonewall Café on Christopher Street in Greenwich Village in May 2001. The café is considered the site where the modern gay movement was born.

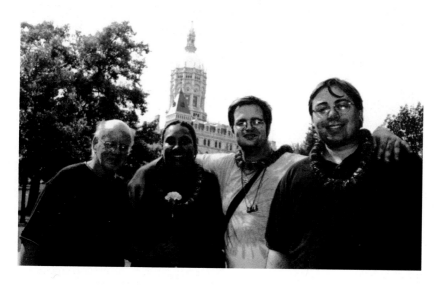

From left to right, Ben, Diane Strong, Andrew, and Will enjoy Connecticut's 2001 Gay Pride Festival on the lawn of the State Capitol in Hartford.

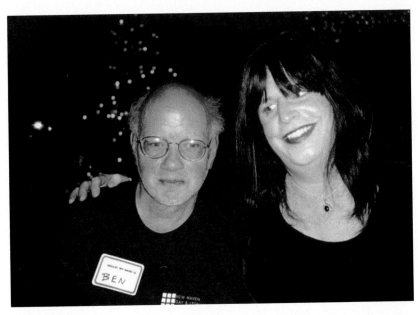

Ben and Lisa became instant new friends during the holiday party in December 1999 at the New Haven Gay & Lesbian Community Center.

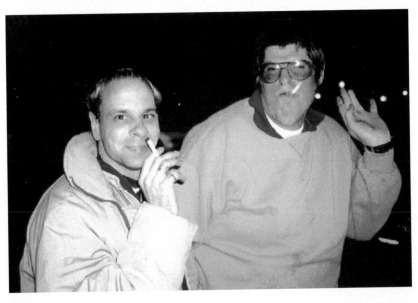

Steven (left) and Bill butch it up while sharing a smoke before a December 2000 meeting.

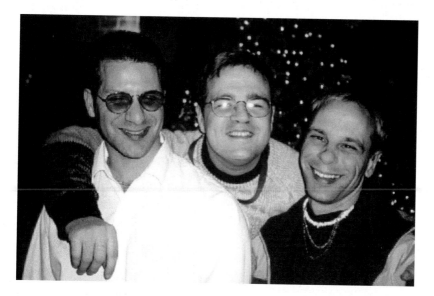

From left to right, Joe, Andy, and Steven share a laugh during the December 2000 holiday party at the New Haven Gay & Lesbian Community Center.

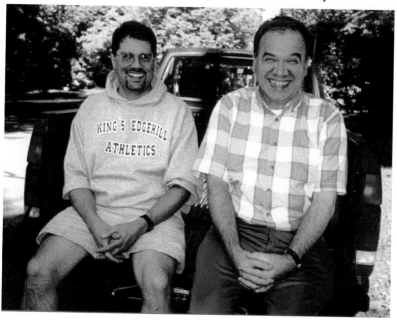

Tim (right) talks about his life story with his friend Peter McKnight outside Peter's house in September 2001. Tim moved to Florida a few weeks after the interview.

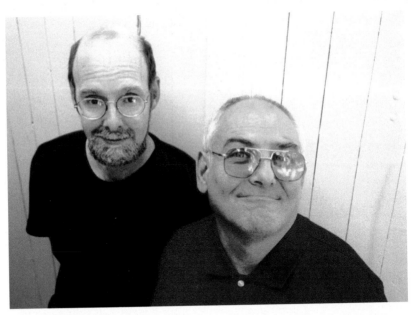

Bob (right) with Denis Caron in September 2001 following Bob's profile interview.

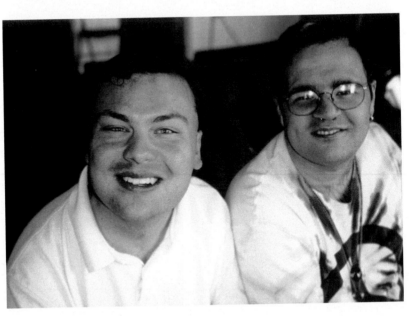

Ron (left) and Andy declare they are boyfriends during the April 2001 meeting at the New Haven Gay & Lesbian Community Center.

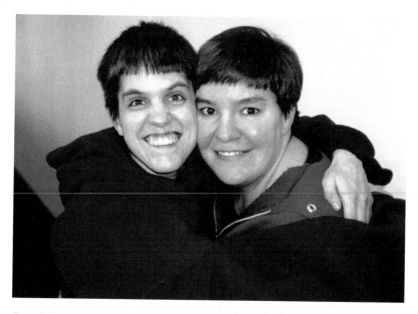

Pam (left) and Dana share a hug. Pam and Dana met in February 2001 and by the April meeting had already declared that they were girlfriends.

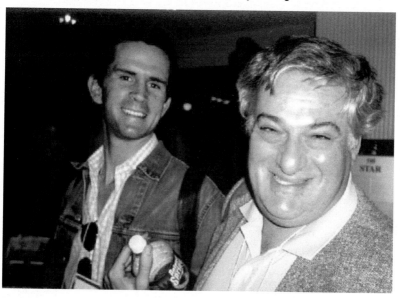

Sean Flanigan, facilitator of a New York City-based support group for gay, lesbian, bisexual, and transgender individuals with developmental disabilities, speaks with Daniel (right) following a May 2002 conference.

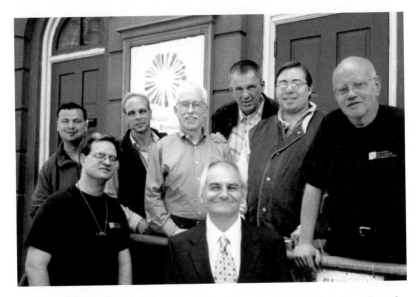

The RSG poses with Robert Woodworth, director of institutional services for the LGBT Community Center in New York City, during a May 2002 sightseeing tour of Greenwich Village.

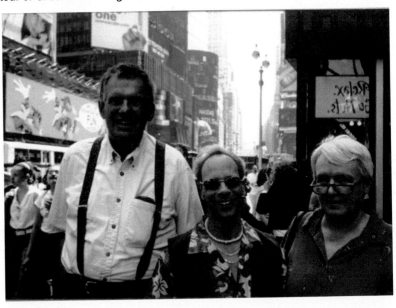

From left to right, Allen, Steven, and Maureen Thomas experience Times Square before speaking at a conference in May 2001.

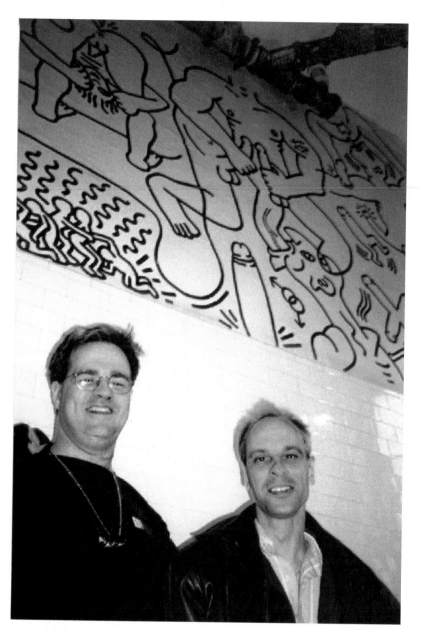

Andy (left) and Steven pose by the Keith Haring mural in a conference room at the Lesbian, Gay, Bisexual, and Transgender Community Center in New York City in May 2002.

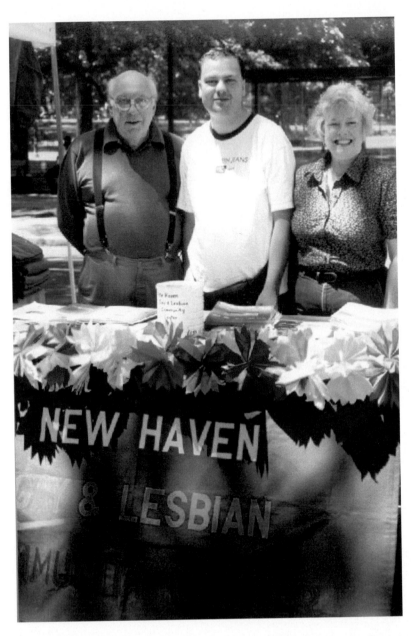

Ron (center) works at the New Haven Gay & Lesbian Community Center information booth with Jack and Betty Allen during the June 2002 New Haven Gay Pride Festival.

# Chapter 7

# Pam and Dana

"What's the best part of getting together?" I asked the two.
"The private stuff," they both answered in agreement.

The love story of Pam and Dana is among the biggest successes of the RSG, but it is also the most difficult to describe. Both women came to the group with a single focus—to find a girlfriend—but their emotions have always remained private and are now reserved for the sanctity of their relationship.

During the first two years of the RSG, Pam was the only lesbian who regularly attended. Group members were puzzled about why women would show up and inevitably not return. As one of the group's founding members, Pam knew who she was prior to attending the RSG. Comfortable in her sexual orientation, she was aware of what she expected from the group and spoke of her desire at every opportunity. Shy and respectful, Pam effectively used the RSG for assistance at her required quarterly and annual support team meetings as reinforcement to remind staff that her primary goal was to find a companion. She eventually met her goal while she was active in the RSG.

The RSG has presented at several conferences during its history. During the meeting prior to the first conference, everyone went around the room and stated the messages they wanted to share with the audience. Pam spoke confidently about her sexuality.

"I like coming to the Rainbow Support Group," said Pam, who was born in June 1970. "I feel comfortable just being in a queer space. I like wearing my community center T-shirts and I even bought new rainbow-colored eyeglasses. Since I am the only lesbian in the group, I hope more women will start attending."

Because of the loneliness she felt as an adult, Pam continually formed deep, emotional attachments with women she saw on a regular basis, who were typically staff and health care workers. During one of the early RSG meetings, she emotionally described her last counseling session during which her therapist told her they could no longer work together. Pam had developed a crush on her therapist, who then decided to end their working relationship. In addition, Pam said the therapist recommended that she have a psychosexual evaluation. Pam expressed fear of a possible behavioral plan.

"I'm afraid my staff are going to try to turn me straight," she said during the February 1999 meeting. The fear was not without merit, since she described previous attempts when staff sought to make her conform to their expectations because they were uncomfortable with her sexuality.

In the spring of 2000, Pam bought a computer and began accessing the Internet. The experience was particularly liberating for her. One of her favorite activities was observing a few of the chat rooms for lesbians. She said she would mostly read the written conversations of others because she felt too self-conscious to join the dialogue. Ultimately, she did manage to connect with someone.

Pam's new partner, who was fourteen years older than her and did not have a developmental disability, lived in another state nearly a day's car ride away. The two began an immediate long-distance and torrid relationship that included daily telephone calls, e-mail love-letters, and at least four visits in which the new partner drove to Pam's condominium for weekends of fun and exploration. The relationship was fully supported by Pam's support team once the partner was sufficiently counseled about the potential liability of getting involved with a person who had a developmental disability. The relationship ended as quickly as it began after six months, no doubt because of the distance.

On January 16, 2001, Pam called me to say she just needed to talk with someone following a telephone conversation she had with her partner the previous day.

"[We talked] and she said she met someone [on the West Coast] and she likes her very much," said Pam, who said she had been crying since the phone call. "She said that because I was in a group home setting I would never get better. She has a plane ticket bought by the new girl and they're getting together February 13, the day before Valentine's Day, and that makes me even madder. This person bought her a plane ticket right before Valentine's Day."

Pam said her partner was traveling to the West Coast to determine the possibility of a relationship with the new woman.

"I never thought about this or [whether] this could happen," said Pam. "I was only thinking about the future. I was happy inside because she was my girlfriend. She was planning to move up here after her son graduates from high school and goes into [military service]."

Toward the end of the conversation, Pam said she was at least glad her partner was honest with her and grateful to have experienced the past six months.

"I mean, it still hurts," said Pam. "This is very upsetting for me. It's not easy, because I really liked her. She was nice. She was a woman. I didn't really find her attractive—she was all right, I guess, but she told jokes."

As fate would have it, at the next meeting, on February 12, 2001, a new woman—Dana—came to the RSG. The meeting was memorable for several reasons, but for Pam it provided closure for her previous relationship just in time for another to blossom. During the meeting, Pam discussed the breakup and said her former partner told her she never loved her, but that they could still be friends—just not girlfriends.

In what stands out as a shining compassionate moment for the group, the other members rallied around Pam and embraced her. One member said that the statement must have been false and suggested the two women must have shared a mutual love. How else could anyone explain the four visits and the daily conversations?

Following the meeting, as members were preparing to leave, Dana approached Pam and the two exchanged e-mail addresses. By the March meeting, the two had already gone on a date, declared their relationship, and made a grand entrance holding hands and wearing smiles that revealed their feelings.

"There's a joke in the lesbian community about what happened with you two," I said to them as they walked into the March meeting. "What do lesbians bring on a second date? A U-Haul. You two fit the mold."

The RSG is not a dating service, but it does provide for the members, and it certainly provided for Pam, a framework where they can take comfort and feel connected to a larger group. Through Pam's involvement with the group, she was able to build her confidence as a lesbian, practice the vernacular of the gay community, and begin to envision a life that matched her feelings. The RSG did not arrange her personal relationships, but the message of the group had been internalized and influenced her interactions with other women.

As a partner, Dana is an even match for Pam. Attractive and aware of lesbian culture, the two women maintain a butch, tomboyish appearance. Both knew from an early age they were lesbians—Dana said she knew at the age of five and Pam said she has always known. Both have developmental disabilities and have wonderfully supportive family members who accept their sexuality and want to support their choices. Both women have also had difficulties in past relationships.

Dana came to the RSG following the breakup of a four-year relationship. She had met a woman in her vocational program and while their feelings were mutual, the woman was not her own legal guardian and still lived in a home where homosexuality was considered taboo. The two were able to experience their relationship only during quick moments seized throughout the workday or secretly when they spent the night at each other's house. The relationship came to an abrupt and traumatic end once her partner's family discovered the clandestine relationship. The breakup resulted in Dana spending months at home, immobilized by depression, so her support team was eager to have her participate in the RSG. Everyone associated with Dana, especially the RSG, was delighted with the news of her budding relationship with Pam. The two became the definitive success story of the RSG and are perceived as role models for the others.

On the May 2 trip to an international conference on DD/MR in New York City, Pam and Dana were inseparable. Oblivious to the world around them, they walked arm in arm on the streets of Manhattan and held hands on the train. They made it clear they did not want to participate in the scheduled activities of the day or spend time with other members. This was their excursion—their own agenda—and they wanted to be only with each other, not the group.

Over the next few months, Pam and Dana became even closer. With deliberate demands to staff and family, they were consistent in their desire to move in together. Staff felt they could begin having overnight visits as a preliminary measure. Pam was permitted to stay over at Dana's family home every Wednesday and every other Saturday. The arrangement was expedited when Dana's monthly phone bill reached $600.

"This is considered a stepping-stone before they move into an apartment together," said Dana's mother, who waited in her car while Pam and Dana said goodbye after returning from the New York conference. Dana's mother was also eager to have her daughter secure an apartment since it was what Dana and Pam wanted.

On November 12, 2001, the two women moved into a cozy one-bedroom apartment in a complex down the street from where Dana grew up. Their apartment was at first sparsely furnished with only a few pieces of furniture—a desk, a bed, and a few donated items. Both enjoyed delineating the chores and gravitated toward favorite domestic duties. Dana cooks and Pam cleans. Pam arranges for her own medications and Dana serves as the spokeswoman for their relationship. With the natural support of Dana's family nearby, as well as both of their support staff teams, the move made sense. They quickly settled into a routine of responsibilities and are clearly living together as a couple.

Once their living arrangements were secured—their goal clearly met—they quickly lost interest in attending the RSG, although neither wanted to formally resign. They had a legitimate excuse for missed meetings though, since transportation was always the biggest obstacle for both Pam and Dana—separately and then after they moved in together. They each had a forty-mile ride to attend the meetings, which was a continuous battle for limited staff and working family members who tried to accommodate various schedules. Once they were in their new living situation, it became even more difficult to arrange rides since Pam left a supported living apartment and Dana moved out of her family home.

"Both are adorable," said Kim Steel, a support staff member who has worked with the couple. "Dana plays strong and Pam plays diminutive."

The two are experiencing the joys and difficulties of what occurs when someone moves into a new apartment. "We don't like having to pay to wash clothes," said Dana, incredulous that the laundry service in the building costs $1.25 per load.

The new situation has provided unforeseen benefits as well. Estranged from her father for most of her adult life—Dana is thirty-five—the father and daughter have rekindled their relationship.

"My father even gave Pam a nickname, 'Minnie'," said Dana, clearly pleased to be honest with her parent. "My father even signed for this apartment."

Two weeks after they moved into the apartment, they said the best part of the experience was spending time together. They did admit that there were a few arguments, but the disagreements were quickly forgotten once they sat down and discussed the problems.

"What's the best part of getting together?" I asked the two.

"The private stuff," they both answered in agreement.

Since nowhere in the United States can two people of the same sex legally marry, the two hope to one day have a ceremony that is similar to a wedding, known as a commitment ceremony. They hope to have a church ceremony, invite family and friends, celebrate with a reception, and then go on a Bermuda cruise for their honeymoon.

"I got engaged to her again," said Dana. "I got down on my knee and asked her to marry me. We're saving our money for a commitment ceremony and a honeymoon."

# Chapter 8

# Steven

"He was a good friend. He was there through everything for me. People can come and go, but me and my dog would be there for each other forever."

A rainbow windsock bounces in the wind next to Steven's front door. The cheerful greeting in the tidy, but otherwise bleak, sixty-unit garden apartment complex, is just one of the overt signs of the person behind the door.

Like emotions on a sleeve, Steven lives his life exactly as the front of his house reveals. A sticker on the mailbox indicates this is the home of Steven and Jeffie. There's a freestanding ashtray separating the front door and a two-seater bench that overflows with Merit cigarette butts. And even though we had a definite afternoon appointment for 3:30, he left his staff and me waiting outside a dark and empty apartment for twenty minutes while he visited with a neighbor. Steven is a complicated personality—described by his staff as manipulative and needy.

Owned by the state of Connecticut, the apartment complex is restricted to senior citizens and people with disabilities. Among the tightly knit group of residents, Steven was the out of place thirty-five-year-old youngster who moved last year into a one-room efficiency apartment. His twelve-by-eighteen-foot apartment sits on the corner of a one-story building housing five other units, each with their own private entrances. Steven's apartment has become a popular focal point for shut-in neighbors desperate for gossip and eager to observe the daily stream of staff who provide residential support. At first unwelcome, Steven has a way of endearing himself toward older people and has since become an integral part of the quiet complex, partly for the entertainment he creates.

73

"At first they thought I was a troublemaker, but now I get along with them," said Steven, who is sociable with many of his neighbors and befriended one who enjoys dogs, which is one of Steven's favorite subjects. "They asked me why there is so much staff."

Steven is "hip," with streaked hair and trendy clothing, but he is always aware that his first presentation to others is as a person with obvious disabilities. He is partially deaf and wears a hearing aid. At five feet, two inches tall and weighing 110 pounds, he has an unsteady gait and walks with a limp. Although he has great language skills and a well-developed vocabulary, the loud nasal tone and unusual quality to his voice contributes to the impression that he is a person with mild mental retardation. A heavy smoker, Steven smokes one to two packs of cigarettes a day and has required assistance to overcome addictions to alcohol and marijuana.

"I have a little limp, a hearing aid, and a speech impediment," said Steven, describing his disabilities. "For that, people would shut me down (waves his arm sideways, pausing to search for the right words), dismiss me. If I didn't have those, maybe I'd have a chance to have a boyfriend."

When Steven describes himself, he often uses self-deprecating descriptions. He envisions himself as a person with disabilities, not as a unique individual with complicated emotions.

"If I describe myself, I would put myself down. I don't really like who I am. I have a lot of staff around. I don't have a boyfriend," he said and then offered the following description of what he would include in a personal ad. "I'm nice to hang out with, but when I get moody, I'm not nice to be with. I'm thirty-five years old, single, gay, white male, looking for someone."

"I sleep a lot," he said, taking a more disinterested tone. "If I don't want people around me, I don't want to be bothered. I turn off the lights and won't answer the door. Often, I do that."

Steven said his goals in life have remained consistent and only their order of importance changes over time. Usually, he is concerned with companionship, securing his own home or condominium, enjoying his pets, and having a job he enjoys and is paid well to do.

When entering his apartment, what's most noticeable is that there is an order to the clutter. The entertainment center in the living area is stocked with videos, CDs, books, and stuffed animals. He says a favorite activity of his is watching movies, especially sad family-themed films. His music collection includes mostly contemporary groups ranging from rock and roll to hip-hop to country. A decorating theme throughout the apartment includes stuffed animals in every nook and images of rainbows on magnets, tapestries, and pictures. There is also a beefcake pin-up poster on a side wall under a mood light. Cozy with gay accents, Steven has woven a comfortable theme throughout his home that reflects a person with many sophisticated interests.

Steven works at a local kennel, which he describes as "a day care for dogs." His primary job is to exercise the canine guests by taking them out for walks and playtime. The job seems tailored specifically for him.

"Having a boyfriend used to be my main goal, but that depends on my mood," he said. "My goal now is to get in a good place, a good job, and to get rid of all the support I get. I don't need all that staff."

The staff assigned to work with Steven spends up to six hours with him every evening. He got himself in trouble several years earlier for public sexual activity and now needs heavy supervision as a requirement for living alone in a supported living arrangement.

"They take me out to go shopping or for medical appointments or out to dinner," said Steven. "They are mostly women staff because if I like the male staff, then I try to get them to become my boyfriend."

With seven days of residential support per week, there are at least six staff members who provide direct support to Steven. Steven says that he does not like to regard the staff as employees, but rather as friends. He is candid about not wanting to associate with other people with disabilities and wants to spend time only with nondisabled people.

"I don't want anyone like me, that is disabled," he said. "Lots of people judge me because I'm under [the supervision of a state agency]. I'll have staff until I die and I ain't too thrilled."

Independence is above all the most important consideration in Steven's life. Although he accepts supervision, he freely admits to directing demeaning and inconsiderate behavior toward staff, especially those he does not like.

"My staff, I don't consider their feelings. I can be cruel. It can be deliberate or unconscious," he said, offering to explain why he frequently argues with staff, but also to justify why he was late for the interview. "I can be sneaky and manipulative. I don't like to answer to anybody."

A common complaint from Steven is that he feels lonely and desperately wants a boyfriend. He has a specific image in mind for a partner and refuses to consider anyone that does not live up to the high ideal. He likes the freshman look: someone eighteen to twenty-five years old, clean cut, handsome, compassionate, fascinating, and, above all, without a noticeable disability. His staff and those within his inner circle have encouraged him to look within the Rainbow Support Group to find someone, since there would be fewer complications in arranging activities between people with disabilities. Although Steven is respectful of the other members in the group, he sees each one's perceived faults and never as potential mates.

Steven said he has had several relationships with nondisabled gay men, and there is at least one long-term relationship in his recent past. The two are not currently romantically involved and have remained platonic friends.

"We were boyfriends seven years ago for two years," said Steven. "He was closeted and too old. He was three years older."

More than any other description, Steven considers himself a gay activist and proudly proclaims his sexual orientation. He has great respect for those who also live an openly gay life.

Steven has an uncanny ability to make others feel sorry for him, which is partly genuine empathy felt for his situation. However, he also is somewhat manipulative. He frequently complains he doesn't have anyone in his life, but what he says and what he does are not always congruent. During the one-and-one-half-hour interview, he fielded five phone calls from friends, a staff person, and a new acquaintance he met through the gay center, all the while complaining about an overwhelming sense of loneliness. With finesse, he expertly maneuvered multiple conversations in the room and over the phone. Even while he was recalling the most intimate details of his past, he was able to arrange dates for socializing, work, and medical appointments. For all of his effort to make the best of his life circumstances, his inability to find inner peace seems rooted in the one condition that will never change, which is that he is a person with multiple disabilities.

Aware of his sexuality at an early age, Steven said he knew he was gay by age ten when he participated in sexual games with friends. He vividly recalled a school friend from the neighborhood where he grew up who Steven engaged in youthful experimental sexual play.

"He taught me a game about sex," said Steven. "We would touch each other."

Steven recalled a much more sinister period of his life, when sexual activities were not welcomed—the ages of fourteen to sixteen. His brother, who was a year older and has since died, was a lifelong drug addict and regularly forced himself on Steven.

"I remember my brother would get high on drugs and cocaine and he would always rape me. He was a little bigger in size," he said.

Steven said his brother never overcame the drug problem and moved to the West Coast when he became of legal age. When he died ten years ago and the body was flown home for the funeral, Steven had a cathartic experience.

"When he died and I was at his funeral, I went up to the casket and started screaming at him, 'Thank God you are dead.' I was so mad at him," he said, explaining that his emotions were involuntary and had poured out of him in a screaming and tearful rage.

Steven said the rest of his family was present and although they never spoke to him about why he was screaming at the funeral, he believed they were aware of the reason for the ill feelings between the siblings.

"I didn't care," said Steven, who added that he told family members when the sexual abuse occurred but was never believed or protected.

Steven said he came out to his father when he was fourteen and the experience was traumatic. "I was fourteen years old and we were in a store and a pack of cigarettes fell out of my pocket. He smacked me and then I told him I was gay, and he smacked me again. My dad doesn't talk, he screams," he said.

Steven described the relationship with his father as guarded. However, during recent years he said the two of them have become more pleasant toward each other and have begun sharing monthly visits.

"I'll never be tight with my father because of my lifestyle and he works too much," he said, explaining that his father has never been comfortable with the knowledge that Steven is gay.

Steven's family is an amalgamation. The youngest of three children by his father's first wife, Steven also has a biological sister four years older than him who lives in a nearby town. His biological parents divorced when he was still a toddler and Steven rarely sees his mother, since she lives in the Midwest. He says that the two are not close.

His father remarried several years after the divorce and the relationship Steven had with his first stepmother was contentious during the four years his father and stepmother were married.

"I didn't like her. We went at it every day, head to head, and my father would stick up for her," said Steven. His stepmother had several other children and Steven said that she did not treat him well.

"She made me stay in my room and favored her children over me," he said.

His stepmother sent him to a school for troubled children in an adjoining state at age fourteen, where he stayed for two years.

"Because she couldn't handle me," said Steven. "I would run away, stay out late. I hit her several times, because she would hit me."

Steven said that when he was twenty, his father married for the third time. He liked his new stepmother and regarded her as the mother he never had and always wanted. Unfortunately, she died a few months earlier and Steven felt a great sense of loss. Steven continues to remain close to her daughter, who lives nearby. The two stepsiblings have developed a close bond, which he says is the most significant familial relationship he has.

Pets can fill an important role in the life of anyone without a partner who has plenty of love to share. For Steven, his beloved snow-white miniature poodle, Jeffie, was a best friend for ten years. Steven has always had pets—dogs, cats, birds, rabbits, guinea pigs—but without question, Jeffie served as a special friend in Steven's life.

"He was a good friend. He was there through everything for me. People can come and go, but me and my dog would be there for each other forever," said Steven, fondly recalling the relationship he had with Jeffie. At fourteen years old, Jeffie died just two months earlier and Steven continues to mourn his friend.

"People, you have to work on the relationship, but dogs are there on bad days, good days, or when you move five thousand times. My dog always went with me wherever I went and that was good. I would jump to get another dog, but my friend said to wait a year," he said.

Never without a pet, the wait to replace Jeffie was too unbearable. Steven went to the local dog pound and paid six dollars for a one-year-old white poodle and beagle mix.

"I named him Jack," he said. "He doesn't bark too much and doesn't jump up."

# Chapter 9

# The Quiet Guys:
# Daniel, Will, Allen, Bob, and George

"I get a lot out of this group," said Daniel. "People talk about their life and their problems. I come here because there are people I could trust that like me. I'd like to become friends with someone and maybe get to come over and stay for a weekend. I'm looking for a boyfriend just to do things with. They can be my age, older, or younger. The person can have a disability."

Many of the people who come to the RSG share similar characteristics surrounding their sexuality. Aware and socially alone in their sexual orientation, they hold conflicting feelings about what they feel inside and how best to display those feelings within society and their personal support network. They are usually dependent on others for much of their daily living requirements and if support staff and guardian family members have an antigay bias, they may intuitively understand that a safe plan of action is to squelch the desire or, in other words, remain in the "closet." Although being in the closet may avoid confrontations with unsympathetic staff or family members, the unacknowledged desire can manifest itself by creating invisible personalities and greater dependency as well as sneaky behaviors that leave the person open to assault, STDs, and emotional turmoil (Savin-Williams, 2001).

After several years and dozens of members coming to the meetings, several personality traits have surfaced. It became apparent that although someone may identify as GLBT, that does not necessarily mean they have acted on those desires. They may be able to articulate their feelings, but that does not indicate they have had gay experiences. A person can be gay without acting on the feelings, just as someone else can be heterosexual without becoming sexually active.

The condition of being gay reveals more about how a person feels inside than about their actions.

The RSG is an appropriate forum for members to connect with others to enjoy a shared gay experience. Although some members may have never acted on their desire, support group meetings and scheduled events serve an important function to bring people together into a queer space where they can at least participate in the community. The interaction serves to validate their feelings, build self-esteem, and counter some of the negative messages they may hold surrounding their sexual orientation. What is truly amazing to observe is the initial reaction when someone new walks into the gay center and realizes a sense of relief to have found a home. Although not everyone will connect with a partner or find a soul mate, participating in a community activity and sharing interactions with others who feel the same way is part of the human experience everyone is entitled to enjoy.

### Daniel

Manhattan is seventy-five miles and a two-hour train ride from the center. Daniel makes the trip once a month with his staff member so he can connect with the RSG and enjoy the company of others who discuss similar concerns. Born in Europe, but raised in the United States, he has lived in a group home in Manhattan since 1973. He feels uncomfortable discussing his sexual orientation in the residence he shares with other developmentally disabled men and women who are not gay. Although he is his own legal guardian and makes his own personal and vocational decisions, his parents and two younger brothers are active and influential decision makers in his life. Daniel, fifty-five, has not always demonstrated good judgment in his quest for companionship and believes that his family has used its influence to ensure that he lives in a supervised setting.

"I would prefer a supported apartment, but my mom preferred me in a group home, because she's afraid I might invite strange people into my apartment," said Daniel, who has not come out to his family. "So, I'm still in a group home. I understand it, but no, I do not accept it. I love my mom—I love her dearly, but I'm angry at her."

Finding a companion is Daniel's primary goal now. He feels overwhelmingly lonely, which was exacerbated by the September 11, 2001, terrorist attack on the World Trade Center where he worked.

During that infamous morning, he reported to work at 8 a.m. at the same agency where he had worked for more than twenty years, and had to flee for his life less than an hour later. The traumatic experience made him realize how alone he feels. Daniel admits to placing himself at risk and making poor judgments in the past regarding his physical and emotional needs. Daniel would like someone to share his life with or, at the very least, to find a partner to go out for an evening, to the movies, or to spend nights at home.

Daniel has fond memories of participating in the activities during Halloween in New York City and is proud of having served as a volunteer during the Gay Pride celebrations in the past through the group, Heritage of Pride, which runs the New York City Gay Pride parade and festival. He is especially dedicated to the RSG.

"I get a lot out of this group," said Daniel, who commutes to RSG by train and taxi. "People talk about their life and their problems. I come here because there are people I could trust that like me. I'd like to become friends with someone and maybe get to come over and stay for a weekend. I'm looking for a boyfriend just to do things with. They can be my age, older, or younger. The person can have a disability. I just want a loving relationship like everyone else."

## Will

Dating and companionship are among the most frequent topics of discussion within the group, but it is always fraught with complications. Even when a member successfully develops a relationship with another person, there are frequent difficulties with obtaining transportation, accommodating staff requirements, and finding a comfortable location for privacy and intimacy.

During the first three years, discussions at monthly RSG meetings focused on the obstructions members had to navigate to move beyond the initial steps of relationship building. A relationship involves feelings of mutual respect, attraction, shared interests, and compromise. Even when members develop friendships beyond the group, they may then have difficulties trying to build and maintain something more meaningful.

Will is a founding member of the RSG, yet his story exemplifies the dilemma facing many members. They desire relationships, but sometimes lack the capacity to build and maintain them. Part of the difficulty is due to their disabilities, but, moreover, I believe their inability to secure and maintain relationships is due to the lack of attention devoted to providing them the skills they need. Only the most sexually active and vocal clients are cautioned about sexual expression. Residential and vocational programs have little room in their budgets or time schedules to dispense information viewed as suggestive by the more conservative factions in the profession.

Prior to the founding of the RSG, Will occasionally made an appearance at the New Haven Gay & Lesbian Community Center for a meeting of the gay men's discussion group. Quiet and observant, Will struggles with his weight and has a high, breathy voice that makes it hard to understand his speech. His behavior both during and after the meetings developed into a predictably uncomfortable routine for the other members. During the few meetings he attended, he refrained from speaking and targeted group members he found attractive with telephone calls and explicit letters. After getting to know Will and understanding how he attempts to connect with others, his actions now seem harmless, but at the time they were off-putting and served only to further ostracize him. It was not until we held the first meeting of the RSG and he attended with staff did his activities become clear.

Will identifies as a gay man, but is someone who has very little gay history. He has never had a boyfriend and has not experienced gay sex. However, having a relationship is his primary goal for attending the RSG and some of the other groups at the center.

"Will's story is very real," said Dr. Maureen Thomas. "Some people are not active on their sexuality, they may not be cute or socially skilled, but they have these feelings and thoughts that are definitely gay."

Thomas said that since the members participate in the group at the center, they at least have an opportunity to experience their sexuality in an affirming environment. Having access to the group, even for only a few hours each month, provides moral support to counter some of the negative messages in society.

"He's not just a guy who has these secret feelings but has a community that helps to validate who he is," said Thomas, who stressed the importance of having the support group meet in a gay-identified meeting space so Will and the other members can at least feel connected to a larger community. "Hopefully, something will come along, but at least for now he has a community."

Further complicating Will's interest in finding companionship is his desire to socialize with people who do not have a disability.

"I want someone not disabled like me. I want someone normal," said Will, thirty, who lives in a supervised apartment supported by an upscale, private, nonprofit residential agency. "I consider myself a little bit normal, but mostly special."

Will said that for him, "normal" is someone with "no physical disability, healthy, no drugs, no smoking, no one with AIDS or in an accident, not married or divorced, someone that looks like Dustin Hoffman, someone that has experienced life."

Will does not have a definitive coming-out story; instead, both he and his family came to know about Will's sexuality over time, particularly during the past few years.

"There was no big event so I'm unclear when he declared his sexuality," explained Will's father, a telecommunications executive consultant. "We were aware when as a teenager—that he shared with the doctors that in his sexual development, he was trying to figure out where he fit in. It was only about four years ago that we began hearing the word 'gay' in his vocabulary."

He said Will is not comfortable in general talking about his emotions and is uncomfortable with this subject in particular.

"We've known he's special and not living a normal life of a thirty-year-old and being gay on top of that, I'm ambivalent about [acknowledging his sexuality]," said Will's father. "My first reaction is that it further complicates an already complicated situation. He is an emotionally fragile person and then there's always the awareness that he has a hard time expressing his feelings in appropriate ways and we fear him getting taken advantage of."

Will's parents, who live in another state in the Northeast, are aware of his explicit letter writing and said the letters are written after he meets someone and wants to express his interest in developing a friendship.

"It's hard from a parents' view to know how to respond," he said. "Why the letter? It's uncomfortable for him to talk directly on a subject that has a lot of feelings and emotions connected. It's very difficult for him."

Will's father explained Will's disability as a learning disability. When Will was a child, his parents did their best to provide good educational opportunities for him.

"Will was labeled learning disabled. He has great difficulty with math and numbers and a typical short attention span," said his father. "And certainly it is complicated with the emotional scars from childhood."

A few days before a scheduled telephone interview with Will's father, I informed Will I had made the appointment with his father. After we spoke, Will left a series of six lengthy and rambling phone messages over the next two days that were mostly inaudible since he talks fast and in a high voice whenever he experiences stress.

The messages began with promises to have better attendance at the RSG meetings and to act more socially appropriate when meeting new men. With each message, Will displayed greater anxiety. He was concerned that my telephone interview with his father would somehow reveal too much personal information which he has not shared with his family. For me, the messages revealed that even though Will's gay life is limited, he is aware of his feelings and trying his best to satisfy a desire for companionship.

The messages, left at various times of the night and early morning over the two days, have been condensed to only include what was clearly understood:

> I appreciate being in the RSG. I want to meet men outside the RSG that are normal.

> When you talk with my dad, tell him I'll see him soon. I really don't want to talk about my dating habits. It's a lot of dirt that shouldn't be rehashed. It's none of his business.

> I hope you can help me meet men this summer. I'd like to get started on that. I don't have any experience. I think the center should have a wealth of men, but there's a shortage and slim pickins'. Also, I'm interested in finding someone to talk to.

Will went on to say he will probably place a personal ad in a publication and was interested in suggestions for what to write and where to place the ad.

> I don't have anyone in my life. I'm not into the bar scene. I don't have any other outlets and I really don't want to [look in my home state].

Following my conversation with Will's father the next day, I called Will to inform him of the content of the interview and to ease his concerns.

"Do they think I'm a failure? I feel like a failure," said Will, interrupting me before I had a chance to begin. "I don't have a job. I'm living off their money. I have no paid employment."

I told Will his father was very understanding of who he is and pleased that he lives in an independent, yet structured, setting. I also shared a vignette his father revealed that speaks to the potential of Will's personality.

"He's an incredibly warm people-person," said Will's father. "He has a remarkable memory about friends and family we haven't seen in years that is absolutely phenomenal and it's a genuine and compensating trait of the disability. He remembers them and will ask about their daughter, a baby, and other details about them. But it's one of the offsetting strengths that is wonderful."

### Allen

Another long-term member of the RSG who is looking for a partner, came to the group with a story much different than Will's. Nearly sixty years old, Allen knew he was gay at fifteen and has acted on his desires when the opportunities were presented. Generally quiet and reserved, he was active in expressing his sexuality as a younger man when his living arrangement afforded him greater freedom.

"I used to meet friends all over," said Allen, who is very friendly and enjoys meeting new people. He said that for years when he was younger, he was able to go out on his own without staff and frequently met men looking for a shared sexual experience. He would arrange to meet them later at their home or in a secluded section of a park. To him, sexual activity was simply part of making new friends and a component of friendship. Once his activities were discovered, they were cause for alarm for those in his support network. He now lives in a supervised group home, under twenty-four-hour supervision.

"I'm looking for a man over forty," said Allen during the train ride to New York City to speak at an international conference on DD/MR. "He must be nice. He can be black, white, brown, Asian—it doesn't matter."

Allen said his partner would have to like the things he enjoys, which are bowling, traveling, and conversation.

"I want the person to like what I like," he said.

Allen is not his own legal guardian and has family members who are actively involved in his life. He said his family is not comfortable with his sexuality, which has been the source of great conflict for him.

"I wouldn't bring my partner around to family functions," said Allen when asked whether he could share that side of his life with his family members. "I don't want to cause troubles."

Allen said his family knows how important the RSG is to him since it provides an important alternative social outlet to the informal network he previously developed. He recognizes that while he is not able to have the same freedom he enjoyed as a younger man, his participation in RSG is a compromise that gives him the opportunity to enjoy a sense of community without assuming the same personal risks.

### Bob

For people with developmental disabilities, there is something comforting about maintaining a connection with a state agency. Even though the residential and vocational programs have dramatically changed within the past two decades, the DD/MR community is still a ghetto. Gone are the massive residential institutions of the mid-1900s, most of which are now closed since residents have been moved into more personalized dwellings. Similarly, the large, private, non-profit vocational programs have evolved into community-focused employment centers. Although the changes profoundly altered the human services landscape, clients are still inalterably connected to the state system.

Bob is someone who has sporadically attended the RSG. Pleasant, with a good sense of humor, he is the master of one-liners. He was born in July 1947, in a small industrial city in Connecticut.

"That was the day hell was born," said Bob, referring to his birthday. "That's what my parents used say."

An incessant talker, Bob is still someone who appears to be invisible. Telling jokes is part of his personality. He opened the first of two interviews with a joke: "I don't drink, smoke, or swear, but goddam it, I just left my cigar at the bar."

Although candid about his relationship and his life, Bob has an old-school mentality when the topic turns to his sexuality. He still shies away from using words that would identify him as gay.

"I don't see my family," said Bob, who is the middle of five children. "My mom has a notion I am gay. I told her once."

Bob describes his childhood as a sad period in his life. His father died in the mid-1980s, having developed cancer from working at a chemical factory. Bob said his relationship with his father, whom he describes as "a drifter and alcoholic," was difficult and abusive. He still harbors tremendous anger toward his father.

In July 1977, Bob met his partner, Vern, who worked mostly as a bookkeeper. Vern did not have a developmental disability but had spent part of his life in a state-run residential hospital for mental illness. (Vern died shortly after our interviews, around Christmas 2001, at the age of fifty-five after a battle with esophageal cancer.)

"I knew I was gay when Vern moved in," said Bob, who added he was first aware of his same-sex attractions at the age of seventeen. "[Vern] took me out of [the state hospital]. I was working in the workshop. He was a patient in the mental hospital."

Eager to talk about his feelings and life history, Bob said he has never pretended to be straight. He has never had a girlfriend and has always been attracted to males his own age.

Bob said he and Vern made a good match since their living arrangement complemented each other. Bob said he does the cleaning and Vern makes the mess. Vern cooks and Bob pays the bills. During the past few years, Vern was unable to work and Bob's paycheck was the only source of income. They both share a love of their four cats: Princess, White Paws, Lucky, and Cuddles.

Bob seems preoccupied with staying out of trouble and is motivated by fear—fear of going to jail, fear of going back to the state hospital, fear of losing his connections with state agencies, and fear of losing his partner.

"If something happens to Vern, I'll be alone," said Bob, who became instantly sad at the possibility of losing his partner.

Bob said he was diagnosed with mild mental retardation—or borderline intelligence—with an IQ of 69 to 70. During the time he spent at the state hospital, he said he was placed in a ward which he said was known as "the retarded ward," for attention-seeking behaviors such as lighting fires, pulling fire alarms, and demonstrating aggressive-compulsive behaviors.

"Just because I have slight mental retardation doesn't give me an excuse to act like a jackass and do dumb stupid things," said Bob as he rambled about the activities that precluded his adult institutionalization. "I'm not actually retarded. I'm just a little slow."

Bob's support staff member, Denis Caron, said Bob takes great comfort in being connected with the DD/MR system.

"It sets boundaries for him," said Denis. "It provides a framework for his life and gives him a connection with others."

In an ironic twist, Bob has worked for the past nine years as a custodian at another state facility. The campuslike setting where he works was originally a state school for troubled boys. The same building where he formerly lived as a rebellious adolescent is now the building he is assigned to clean. The memories of that tumultuous period in his youth continue to haunt him, yet it was his choice to work at the site.

"It was hard to go back there at first, but the folks were nice to him and he decided to stay," said Denis.

Bob clearly sees himself as partnered and takes pride in that identification. He describes his life as "half of an old married couple." He has a vivid memory of meeting his partner, and he described the moment as surreal.

"Something told me inside that he was the right person for me, like everything stopped for a split second and a voice told me 'This man is for you,'" said Bob with a calm satisfaction that demonstrated pride in his long-term relationship. "My coming out was when I moved in with my friend in 1977."

Bob said he secured a pass to leave the institution for an afternoon into town and went to the YMCA where Vern was living. Bob considers the afternoon rendezvous their first date, where they kissed, made love, and talked.

"I guess it was our first date," said Bob. "He asked me and I said, 'I'd be very honored to live with you.'"

### George

The RSG is not always well received. Usually, if someone feels the group is inappropriate for him or her, the individual may attend only one or a few meetings and then stop, but one of the more unusual episodes occurred with a man who attended from a great distance.

George (an alias) attended the group for almost a year. As he became more comfortable interacting with others at the meetings and at the center, he also became more candid in describing the characteristics of the men he wanted to connect with, which were specifically large, masculine-looking, bearded men. At each meeting, he would bring explicit literature that advertised magazines featuring the type of men he described. He was also sexually active and mentioned he enjoyed coming to the group since he was lonely and the group was a better alternative than meeting strangers in public areas and inviting them home for the evening.

As dedicated as George had become to the group during the first year, he abruptly stopped attending. On several occasions, I called his staff and after a few months, was finally given a response.

"George does not want to attend the group," they said. "He has met someone and feels that the relationship satisfies his social needs."

I told the staff person that I certainly understood, especially since he had to travel a great distance to attend, close to 100 miles each way. I was genuinely excited to hear about his new partner.

"What is his name?" I asked, envisioning a companion that fit George's explicit description.

"Oh, it's not a man. It's a woman. He met a woman and that seems to satisfy his needs. You can keep him on the mailing list, but unless something changes he won't be coming to the group," they said.

Incredulous, I wondered to myself if there was another story behind George's decision to connect with a woman. Was it perhaps that he was merely conforming to the expectations or manipulations of a disapproving agency and staff, or was it a decision contemplated on his own?

Over the next two years, George received the regular mailings and an occasional telephone message reminding him of upcoming meetings. As members have left the group, they may or may not continue to receive the regular mailings that are sent two to three times per year on average. If someone wants to end participation, his or her decision is respected, since the purpose of the group is to help people feel more comfortable with their feelings.

For George, his connection with the group was severed following a telephone message he left regarding a general RSG mailing.

*August 24, 2001, message*

"John, I'll refer you not write me anymore. I got another letter in the mail and my staff member did, too. If you write one more letter, I'm gonna have to call the police. OK? Because this is not good. This is [harrassment].

"I told you many times I didn't want you to write to me or call me. You haven't been calling me, but you've been writin' to me again. I'll refer you not to write anymore, or I'm gonna have to do something about it. OK? And I will call the police, and tell them that you're writing to me and you're [harrassing] me. All righty? So there better be no more letters in this mailbox. OK? My name is [George] and that address you got is [address]. I'll refer you not to do that anymore. OK?

"I have a wife. I'm married. I got married [this year]. All right? And I'm very happy with her, and I'm not gay anymore. OK? So I'll refer not you to call me anymore or write to me.

"You've been doing—you been doing good about the calling, but don't write to me anymore, please. Again, and that's that. All right? All right. Bye-bye."

I called George's staff to hear an explanation about why he would leave such a severe and threatening message, but also about his decision to marry and partner with a woman. The staff person shared little more than what was given two years earlier, which was that George stopped coming to the meetings when he met a woman, who is now his wife. After we established there was miscommunication in removing George's name from the group's roster, the conversation ended with a complaisant request to keep the agency informed through future mailings.

The experience with George and his staff was unfortunately one of the tangible examples that demonstrates the vulnerability for those working with people with disabilities. The legal and ethical implications that will inevitably arise when considering issues as complicated as sexuality, such as those raised by George in his message, serve as a caution to advocate for only those individuals who ask for assistance. George and his agency's contacts were promptly purged from the roster as a preventive measure, along with others who had stopped attending. There is enough literature and flyers disseminated throughout the region should anyone want to reconnect with the group.

I believe that sexuality is not a choice but an organic condition (Bernstein, 1995). The only choice individuals have is whether to be honest with what is going on inside of them. The response I have for George is that he can no sooner change from being gay to straight than he can change what he did during the year he participated in the group. He can, however, choose to conform to the pressures he may feel imposed on him either by society, his support network, or family and friends, but all that does is trade one repressed sexuality for another.

I respect George's decisions and share in his struggle for personal acceptance. For anyone who has ever questioned his or her sexuality, it is an arduous journey to find inner peace and, for some, can take a lifetime to complete. Although I respect his choices, I also know the work being done to provide appropriate and safe opportunities for other RSG members has been embraced only tenuously by the profession. As the human services profession struggles to find ways to support the developmentally disabled community in its desire for healthy sexual expression, and one that includes GLBT people, the best hope for George and others in his predicament is to build and enhance a support network around those who have already done the personal work to accept themselves. There is a self-fulfilling prophecy that as more people come out and declare their sexuality, it will be easier for others to do the same.

# Chapter 10

# Bill

"I have something to tell you about my life—my gay life."

Some people can whittle away time telling stories that seem to be about nothing at all. For anyone paying attention, there can be a message derived from the stream of consciousness that offers a glimpse of the personality waiting to surface.

At first glance, Bill could be dismissed as an overweight, goofy chatterbox. More than social chitchat, he produces an incessant chatter to fill the silence around him. In an instant, he can offer reports of current events, personal stories, and unsolicited opinions on whatever happens to cross his visual path.

Observant, quick-witted, and curious, Bill likes to move about the grocery superstore where he works as a bagger and cart retriever like a cat on the prowl. With stealthy ease, he can move a line of carts into the store, pause to share a quick smoke with a fellow associate, and stop to bag groceries and chat with an acquaintance he spots at one of the checkout aisles. The job offers him a continually refreshing landscape filled with anticipation around every corner and regular rounds of customers who enjoy his visits and gossip. With more than five years of dedicated service, Bill is well suited to the job and equally appreciated for his perfect attendance.

Bill said he always knew he was gay and is matter of fact about being sexually active from an early age.

"I had sex with everyone down the street," he said speaking about the many experiences he had during his adolescence.

As young teenagers, he and a best friend had a paper route together for two years and would reserve time along the route for experimenting with sex in apartment hallways or his friend's house, which mostly involved touching each other.

During an interview, accompanied by his long-term vocational support staff member Chris Kapinos, Bill described a childhood that was filled with sexual experimentation. Most experiences were consensual, but some were not. "I had sex with neighbors, cousins, [house] painters, my uncle," said Bill. He described two early sexual relationships he experienced with extended family members. When Bill would visit his grandmother's house in the suburban town where he grew up, a relative close in age was also a frequent guest.

"We would go upstairs in my grandmother's house when she wasn't around," recalled Bill about the experiences that occurred around the time he was twelve or thirteen years old.

Bill said he continues to see his relative, and during a visit last year, the relative, who is now married with children and lives in another state, apologized to Bill for the youthful experiences.

"He visited last year, came to me, and said, 'I'm sorry I did that to you since you're retarded,'" said Bill, who quickly modified the description of himself. "He said, 'I'm sorry, I shouldn't have done that because you're handicapped.'"

"I told him, 'I don't have any problems with what happened and that we were just kids,'" said Bill, adding that he does not dwell on the past and in fact enjoyed the youthful experiences.

What he adamantly did not enjoy were the advances an alcoholic uncle made when Bill was fourteen years old. Bill said that on several occasions, his uncle came into the bedroom where Bill was sleeping and forced himself on Bill.

"It was creepy," said Bill. He never told anyone until recently, when he told his relative, who replied that the uncle, who died in the mid-1980s, had also approached other family members.

"I don't let things bother me," said Bill summarizing his feelings about the unwanted advances.

Bill comes across as a nervous person and seems to relish in obnoxious behaviors. He is overweight and a heavy smoker. He habitually rocks back and forth whether sitting or standing, and whether quiet or engaged in conversation. He often plays with the upper dental plate inside his mouth with his tongue, flipping it over his lips and back in again. He has no qualms about reaching out to touch something of interest on the person in front of him. His frequent laughs are boisterous and over the top, misplaced, and deliberately attention-getting. At functions where there is food, he will eat to excess and then make no effort to conceal a snack load he's placed in his pockets for later. With masterful precision, Bill can embellish his disabilities simply to be annoying, often to his advantage.

Bill is streetwise and has had to be for many reasons. He is first a person with a disability and accustomed to being preyed upon by people. Like so many others with disabilities, he relies on public transportation and walking to get around, which can leave him vulnerable to the urban environment. His loud and abhorrent techniques have proved useful as a deterrent to being victimized, which he rarely is for someone who takes great risks.

Bill has many likable qualities. Honest and candid, he can be generous with his money, possessions, and emotions. Inquisitive and adventurous, he displays an aura of innocence that belies the many sexual conquests he has experienced in his pursuit of companionship. Aided by his involvement in the RSG, he has been able to come out to his co-workers and important support staff, which has had a calming and maturing influence on his public presentation.

Bill revealed that when his younger sister found out that he is gay, it was more traumatic for both of them than he lets on. Nervously laughing when describing the incident, Bill said his sister walked in on him while he was having sex with an anonymous partner he picked up at a local movie theater. Bill said he frequents some of the notorious gay cruise spots on a weekly basis and likes to bring men back to his apartment for the evening.

"I brought a man home from [the movie theater] and [my sister] walked in on us," said Bill speaking louder and becoming more animated. "I forgot to lock the door and [my sister] walked in and found us together."

Bill lives above his sister in a garden apartment development. The two siblings are emotionally close, but Bill had never shared with her that he is gay. He said his sister ran out of the room and the two have never discussed the incident since it happened.

Bill is fully aware of his sexual orientation. He said he likes men because they are "stronger and huskier" than women and revealed his ideal partner would look like Tom Selleck, the actor. Although he accepted his sexuality long ago, he also knows homosexuality is still taboo and he is extremely guarded about what he reveals to others.

"I don't act gay at work. I act gay when I'm by myself," said Bill, explaining that he does not want his co-workers to know he is gay. He is especially careful about displaying stereotypical behaviors around his co-workers such as feminized hand gestures, body movements, and voice inflections.

At work, he said customers and co-workers do not call him derogatory words, either for his disabilities or sexual orientation.

"There's no name calling," he said. "I've been lucky."

I typically shop at the same grocery store where Bill works. When he sees me at the store, it's a trigger for him to begin talking about being gay. One recent exchange occurred when Bill saw me approach the checkout line during a crowded early evening and came over to bag my groceries.

At first he said to the young, friendly female cashier, "This guy runs a group I go to. It's a gay group. He's gay, and I go to this group. And I'm gay."

The moment was filled with tension, humor, and revelation. The cashier responded, "Billy, we already knew you were gay."

"Bill, did you just come out to your co-worker?" I asked. "Are you ready to start coming out to people here at work? Because that's what you're doing."

In a voice intended for more than just the three of us, Bill said loud enough for the dozens of customers and employees to hear within several checkout aisles, "John, when are we going to get together to talk about the book? I've got something to tell you about my life—my gay life."

He accentuated the word *gay,* and began laughing with his typically loud and boisterous laugh.

Bill said he has never had a boyfriend or long-term partner, but he has been friendly with a man since 1990 who works for a local newspaper as a delivery associate. The two met at a well-known gay cruise district along New Haven's waterfront, known as Long Wharf, and have remained friends, or at the very least sexual partners. They get together every few weeks at the man's house. Bill describes him as "tall, thin, and gray hair."

"We get together just to have sex," said Bill. They do not have an emotionally intimate life together, but the arrangement obviously satisfies Bill's needs for companionship.

Bill has a computer and has recently discovered that he can meet other men in chat rooms. "I tell them that I work and I'm sociable. I ask them, 'How old are you? What town do you live in? And can I call you?'" said Bill, who added he gives his name and a description of himself as "tall and a good person looking for someone for sex."

Toward the end of the interview, Bill became deeply thoughtful. He said he knew he did not choose his sexuality and is trying to be more comfortable living openly as a gay person. He called the Rainbow Support Group "wonderful," and noted it has helped him and others feel more comfortable with their sexuality.

"Homosexuality, that's OK, isn't it?" he asked calmly and introspectively. "When we die, we go to heaven and that's where my soul will see that it's OK."

After the interview, Bill's support staff member, Chris Kapinos, said what Bill revealed was at the same time both expected and surprising.

"It's what I expected from him. Bill never told me he was gay, but I've heard it from others," said Kapinos.

Kapinos said Bill is the type of person who enjoys talking, although there is not always a point to his conversations.

"He talks and says nothing as opposed to others that talk and tell stories," Kapinos said.

Kapinos has worked with Bill for ten years and confirmed that Bill is streetwise beyond his disability. Although Kapinos was surprised to hear about some of the incidents in Bill's life, he also questioned whether Bill was sincere in sharing details of his personal life.

"Maybe he's not telling all about himself, but maybe that's all there is," he said, adding that Bill can be guarded and calculating in what he will reveal. "He is a very private person and he may have only told you what he wanted you to hear."

# Chapter 11

# Tim

GWM, 40, handicapped, looking for companionship/lover under 50, handicapped or not. Likes gardening, travel, and camping.

Gay bars have historically been among the few safe gathering spots for gay people, where in addition to serving spirits and friendship, they also serve as a place of refuge and even something resembling a community center (D'Emilio and Freedman, 1997). For more than thirty years, Tim built his life around a local gay bar located a few blocks from his home.

Westport, Connecticut, is known almost as much for its suburban culture and nightlife as it is for some of its famous citizens. At just under an hour's train ride outside of New York City, the liberal-leaning, suburban town is home not only to many celebrities, including Joanne Woodward, Paul Newman, and Martha Stewart, but also to a notorious gay watering hole.

The Cedar Brook Café is a historic establishment noted as the second oldest continuously operated gay bar in the country. Tim became a weekend fixture there the moment he became of legal age to find camaraderie and develop a sense of community. Like so many other gay people, he made a beeline for the café the day he turned twenty-one, and described the place as a second home.

Tim has an easygoing personality and a quick and hearty laugh, which is infectious to those around him. Sociable and honest with his feelings, he was always aware that as a person with a disability, he would not be considered one of the popular patrons at the bar. However, that never sidelined an eagerness to be with other gay men and experience a joie de vivre.

An only child, Tim has a good relationship with his mother, Milly. Milly has always been comfortable with the knowledge her son is gay and has never tried to squelch his desire to develop the private side of his life. Even though she can be protective of her disabled son, Milly has allowed Tim the freedom to have his own feelings. She knew where he went on Saturday nights, but the only rule was that he would have to return home at a reasonable time, which was usually around midnight or one o'clock.

Members participate in the RSG with the assistance of staff who either bring them to meetings or help arrange transportation or other supports. Since Tim is not connected with a state agency, his participation is coordinated with the assistance of his friend, Peter McKnight, a hospital nutritionist who lives near Tim. The two met at the Cedar Brook Café in 1985 and have enjoyed a solid friendship since then.

"We met at the Cedar Brook one night and he asked if we could be friends," recalled Peter. "We discovered that we shared a similar history. Tim grew up down the street from where my mother lived. I empathized with him saying that he had no friends, and it reminded me of growing up not being popular. We moved a lot when I was younger and I had a hard time making friends, so he asked and I accepted to be his friend."

Tim does not have mental retardation, although Milly at first thought he did. Born in February 1949, it was not until he was thirteen that she took him to a research hospital, where a hearing test revealed he was partially deaf.

Through a series of mistakes, Milly and the local school system regarded Tim as mentally retarded, even though he has an IQ of between 85 and 100, and enrolled him in a kindergarten class with other children who had developmental disabilities. This early misstep, along with his hearing loss, set a course for Tim's life that funneled him into a state institution and subsequently into nonprofit vocational programs in the region.

Tim never developed a relationship with his biological father. Milly said Tim's father was unwilling to get married. Tim's father eventually fathered two other daughters and a son, but Tim has never met his half siblings, does not know where his father currently lives, and has had only a few uneventful visits with him.

When Tim was two, Milly married a man she described as alcoholic; the relationship quickly disintegrated. With the divorce finalized two years later, she married her second husband, Alfred, when Tim was four. Although that marriage lasted until Alfred died forty-four years later, there was little cohesion among the three.

"Al didn't get along with Timmy," said Milly matter of factly. "Al was usually very easygoing, but he never treated Tim well. The only problems we ever had revolved around Tim. He mentally and emotionally abused Tim."

For example, Milly said Alfred would severely punish Tim if a scuffle erupted when they visited other friends with children, regardless of what happened.

"Al would immediately slap him. He was always ready to punish him," said Milly, who said both she and Alfred were quiet people. She never understood why Alfred did not like his stepson.

"Even he couldn't explain it," she said.

Sitting for an interview at his friend Peter McKnight's house one late summer afternoon, Tim vividly recalled a much more sinister memory.

As newlyweds, Milly and Alfred lived in a third-floor apartment from 1954 to 1955 above the Bridge Café in the center of Westport. When Tim went out to play in the backyard one day, he was accosted in the back hallway by a patron from the bar, who also happend to be one of Alfred's buddies.

"He pulled my pants down and fondled me. He hurt my penis. He tried to force himself inside me," explained Tim, who said he escaped by pushing himself away from the man when Alfred appeared in the hallway and witnessed what was occurring between his drinking buddy and stepson. "I told him his friend molested me, but [my stepfather] told me, 'Keep your mouth shut or I'll beat the life out of you,'" he said.

Tim said not only did Alfred not come to his defense, Alfred also indicated the incident was appropriate punishment for a misbehaving child.

"He had been drinking, came out of the bar, saw the man hurting me, and said I egged him on. He said that I was a bad boy and said, 'That will straighten you out.'"

Traumatized, Tim said he tried to tell his mother right after it happened, but she could not understand what he was saying.

"It's still very upsetting," said Tim. "I call it rape. I try to get it out of my mind."

Tim was finally able to tell his mother about the incident several years ago, about a year before Al died of heart failure in 1997. In some unexplainable cathartic moment, Tim was able to confront his stepfather about the mistreatment—the pain he endured from years of physical and emotional abuse—and also about the incident at the bar when his stepfather refused to comfort him.

"I asked him why he treated me that way and he did say he was sorry and asked for forgiveness," said Tim, who was unable to elaborate further about why the exchange occurred, saying only that his stepfather had become ill from heart disease.

"Tim reconciled with Al toward the end," said Milly. "I don't know why."

Tim said he began to understand his sexual orientation during early adolescence. At fourteen, he was sent to live at a state residential institution and school, which was considered a national model for people with disabilities. Tim has only fond memories of going to school and making friends during the four years he lived in the institution's rural campus-like setting. He said he made lots of friends and enjoyed the food. He added there were plenty of opportunities to socialize with other residents and said he especially enjoyed the dances held every Friday evening.

Shortly after he arrived at the school, Tim said he had his first sexual experience in one of the residence halls for boys. The experience was with one of the other residents, a large male three years older than him, who was deaf and mute. The experience took place in the resident's bedroom.

"He started to show me himself upstairs," said Tim about his first same-sex experience. He added that he enjoyed the feelings it stirred inside of him, even though he felt too self-conscious to ejaculate. "He pulled his pants down and took my pants down and he started to show me how to shoot. He hugged me after."

Tim recalled how the sexual play quickly became an almost everyday occurrence during the four years he spent at the school. Although he named six other housemates among his regular partners, he said many other boys at the residence routinely participated in mostly masturbatory sexual activity. He said he was never coerced to participate in the activity and that occasionally the boys would touch each other.

"We always agreed," said Tim, referring to the popular group activity.

The activity usually occurred around bedtime and the boys were careful not to be discovered by staff. Tim said staff did not participate in the activity and that he was never approached for sex by staff, even though he was aware other residents had been approached. As a young gay male coming of age, Tim described his residency at the school as an idyllic community where he had friends, sexual partners, and developed his sexual identity and a positive self-image. He has only fond memories of those four years.

In retrospect, Milly said she always knew her son was gay, but her understanding of his sexual orientation occurred only gradually. She knew about some of Tim's sexual escapades since he has never been one to keep secrets from her. She has also come to learn about some of the notorious incidents at the school, but said bad things did not happen to her son. They are both pleased with the treatment he received at the school.

Milly and Tim never had good luck working with the nonprofit rehabilitation agencies in their region. Many of the jobs Tim had were entry-level restaurant and custodial jobs he found on his own. His stepfather, Alfred, a custodian for a local school system for thirty-five years, got him a job for a brief period as an evening custodian at a town school, but he has never participated in long-term employment. Tim is currently unemployed and spends most of his time as a companion for his mother, watching television, and visiting family and friends.

Tim has never really had an official boyfriend, although he speaks candidly about his desire to find a companion. Pointing to his friend Peter McKnight, he said he would like to find someone exactly like McKnight to be his partner, but he is also comfortable enough with himself to say he would be happy to find someone else with a disability.

"I'd like to find someone like me to pal around with and get an apartment," said Tim.

McKnight said he is surprised Tim has not found a partner, since Tim is certainly not shy about meeting others. However, McKnight indicated it can be difficult for people with developmental disabilities to overcome the stigma of their disability, especially in a competitive and image-conscious nightclub setting.

"Tim has a good sense of humor," said McKnight, who describes his relationship with Tim as both friend and mentor. He said the two of them get together every other month for an afternoon of hiking or going to the Cedar Brook Café, where they talk and share some laughs. "I love making him laugh."

McKnight recalled one of their visits, when he took Tim to see the 1987 gay-themed movie, *Maurice*.

"I took him to see the movie and he was so moved; it was such a big advertisement for having a lover," said McKnight. "It showed two men that had a relationship and you don't know if they're going to make it until the end. There's that whole uncertainty in a relationship, that you so want it, and it moved Tim to see two men have a relationship, a good relationship."

Milly said she will support Tim's decision to find a boyfriend, although he has not been very vocal to her about his dream. She also indicated that just like any concerned parent, a potential partner must be thoroughly scrutinized, especially during this age of AIDS, but that she has no problems about her son living in an openly gay relationship.

"I know some people are different, but I'd have to check the guy out first," she said in a playful yet serious tone.

The closest Tim has come to having a partner was about ten years ago, when he was actively engaged in a search. With McKnight's assistance, he placed his one and only personal ad in a Connecticut gay newspaper, *Metroline*, which read:

> GWM, 40, handicapped, looking for companionship/lover under 50, handicapped or not. Likes gardening, travel, and camping.

The ad proved successful and Tim connected with a man he described as four years older than him who was a technical engineer at a large manufacturing company.

"He was dark-haired and came up to here on me," said Tim drawing a line across his shoulders to indicate his boyfriend's height. Their dates always revolved around the bar on Saturday nights.

"We would have dinner next door at the diner—he would treat—and we would go to his car behind the Brook," said Tim who said that the two were together for about a year. The routine of their dates included dinner, hanging out in the bar, and having sex in the car.

After only six months of participation in the Rainbow Support Group, Tim moved to Florida with his mother to be closer to some of her family members. Tim treated the move as an adventure and was looking forward to new surroundings. For his last weekend in Connecticut, the owners of the bar gave their "old-timer" a send off party with cake and gifts.

"People treated me like family," said Tim, who was obviously touched by their thoughtfulness. "They had a cake and hugged me and everyone was nice to me. They congratulated me and wished me well."

# Chapter 12

# Ben

---

HELP WANTED: Developmentally disabled, heterosexual male, 55, cross-dresser, seeks a part-time personal assistant, up to 20 hours a week, $15/hour, 52 weeks a year.

Responsibilities include assisting with budgeting and domestic responsibilities, scheduling appointments, transportation, take weekly grocery shopping, and especially—making sure his alter ego looks fabulous!

---

While companionship is a primary topic of discussion with RSG members, Ben is interested in developing a different kind of relationship. Ben is a fifty-five-year-old man who identifies himself as heterosexual. He lives on his own in a suburban town, holds a job in the food service industry, recently split from his girlfriend when she moved to another state, and has borderline mental retardation. He is also a longstanding member of the RSG and his participation is appropriate because he is also part of the sexual minority community. Ben has cross-dressed for at least forty-five years and only recently since joining the group has he been able to feel a sense of satisfaction with the activities he enjoys at home—and alone.

By definition of his cross-dressing, Ben is a member of the transgender community. He enjoys dressing in traditional female clothing as a recreational activity. He owns and wears several dresses, wigs, heels, blouses, undergarments, and makeup, and especially indulges in his desire for stockings. Until recently, Ben was only able to experience his alter ego in the privacy of his own apartment—never in public or in the presence of another person. He has endured years of condemnation from unsympathetic staff. His cross-dressing has been used against him as a threat to manipulate his behavior, as fodder for humiliation, and as justification for psychotherapy and even psychotropic medication. Prior to the RSG, no one ever explained to him that cross-dressing was something people have been doing for millennia.

Ben was an active member of the RSG for three years before his support staff found him a personal assistant who understood his unique situation. The hiring process took only two weeks and Ben was able to participate in the interviews. In a bold move, Kim Steel, a support staff member assigned to Ben, assisted in constructing an employment advertisement that ran in the *NHGLCC News* July/August 2001 newsletter:

> HELP WANTED: Developmentally disabled, heterosexual male, 55, cross-dresser, seeks a part-time personal assistant, up to 20 hours a week, $15/hour, 52 weeks a year.
>
> Responsibilities include assisting with budgeting and domestic responsibilities, scheduling appointments, transportation, take weekly grocery shopping, and especially—making sure his alter ego looks fabulous!
>
> Hours are very flexible, but do include 2-3 weekend social nights per month. Mileage and expenses are also covered. Knowledge of diabetes helpful.
>
> Candidate must have a sense of humor, be comfortable with transgender issues, and be sensitive to the needs of a person with a developmental disability.
>
> Anticipated start date, August 1, 2001.

"Ben was assigned to a broker because it was thought that his rights were being violated and that he needed a more individualized and creative approach to allow him to express himself," said Steel. "He wanted less staff involvement and more privacy because he was not happy with how he was being handled. The [state agency] acknowledged that Ben needed this support."

Steel said initially there was tremendous resistance to the changes anticipated in Ben's supervision, primarily from colleagues acquainted with Ben's situation, but she was adamant something needed to change.

"There was a lot of resistance when I first took over Ben's case from his previous team, but Ben was insistent on no longer having [state agency] staffing and he wanted private supports," said Steel referring to the shift from state employees providing residential supervision for Ben to hiring a private individual for his support staff.

"The first thing I asked him was who he wanted in his circle of support, which are the people important in his life that he identifies, rather than an assigned group of staff. He said he wanted [a behaviorist] Maureen Thomas, his therapist, and myself, his case manager, because we were the only people he trusted. The former team was upset that they weren't involved in the process, but I was insistent on validating Ben's wishes," she said.

Once the advertisement was published, Ben's new support staff person was quickly hired.

"Ben hired me," said Meoshia McClendon, who sat in Ben's apartment looking over at him as she described the first time they met. "He interviewed me. He said he wanted me to be on time and understand his lifestyle—the cross-dressing."

McClendon explained that while she was comfortable with Ben's desire to cross-dress, she was also aware the core function of the job was to assist him with his daily living requirements.

"He said he needed his bills paid, someone to help him manage his money, take him food shopping, help him with house cleaning and his hygiene. I'm big on that," she said, referring to personal hygiene. "These are all the things you need to be a responsible person."

Ben said that after only three months, he and McClendon have developed a comfortable working relationship based on mutual respect and genuine friendship. "She's more pleasant, more kind. It offers me more independence," said Ben.

"Independence" and "leisure clothes" are some of the code words Ben uses to refer to his cross-dressing activities. Since Ben's desire to cross-dress developed in tandem with condemnation, he learned early on the activity required secrecy. He has been able to enjoy cross-dressing experiences only during brief moments when he was left unsupervised or when an understanding staff member looked the other way and allowed Ben a moment of privacy. His metamorphosis into another gender has also been self-taught and is, at best, unpolished. With a heavy beard that is usually unevenly shaved and an insistence on smoking cigars, Ben's presentation lacks the sophistication he wants to achieve.

"Barbara, as a person, was created in [February 2000]," said McClendon as she looked over to Ben, who nodded his head in agreement. McClendon did not begin working with Ben until July 2001 but has been able to develop a time line of events based on Ben's descriptions and his participation in the RSG.

"She didn't come out," added Ben, speaking for his feminine personality and making clear that Barbara has never made a public appearance. "She's always been there [inside of me], but she never came out."

Ben owns dresses that he either purchased at a local consignment shop or were given to him by family members or supportive staff. Ben is adept at dressing from the neck down as female, but has never had assistance with completing the experience around his face and hair to create a realistic feminine portrait.

His first experience naming his alter ego occurred during the February 2000 meeting of ConnecticuTView, a group for men who cross-dress that meets at the New Haven Gay & Lesbian Community Center. This first meeting was an opportunity for Ben to be tutored in the unique circumstances surrounding cross-dressing. Lisa, the facilitator of the group, recalled the first few meetings with Ben.

"I first met Ben in December 1999 at the holiday party," said Lisa, a male-to-female cross-dresser who recalled the first meeting with Ben. "At first I didn't know what to make of him. He was in 'male mode.' I saw a retarded and slow person, but I also heard he was transgender. I thought it was terrific because I saw that I could help him."

Lisa said Ben's "radio" was strong, a metaphor akin to tuning an AM radio late at night. The signal contains distortion and varying qualities of reception. "Mostly it is faint and flickering where you can be female for an hour, but it is not permanent," said Lisa, adding that support groups assist men who cross-dress with becoming more comfortable in social settings as their female personality.

During summer 2001, with the anticipated changes in his residential supports, Ben became noticeably more empowered in describing his cross-dressing desires. However, he displayed some obvious confusion when speaking for both Ben and Barbara, exemplified in the following telephone messages:

*June 7*

"Hi, John. This is Benny calling. The reason I'm calling is Barbara doesn't know what to wear for the next—for October fourteenth. That's a Sunday," said Ben referring to the third annual RSG open house on October 14, 2001, which was open to prospective members throughout the region.

Unsteady with alternating between his identities, Ben is still learning to speak for his new personality. "She doesn't know what to wear so why don't you give her a call, give me a call, and I can talk to her about that. So call me if you can, John. Thank you. Bye."

*June 10*

"Hi, John. This is Benny calling. Barbara wants to, Barbara's already talked to [Kim Steel] to see if they can find her some clothes to wear. I don't know what's she gonna wear, but hopefully, she'll wear something nice. So, if you want to give her—give me a call and we can talk about it and see what we could get her to wear. So call me at my apartment tomorrow. So if you get a chance, give me a call. If I'm not here, leave it on my answering machine, John, OK? Thank you. Bye. By the way, John, I'm still going to that—Barbara's still going to go to that thing, Sunday, October fourteenth. All right? So she'll be there, all right? Thank you. Bye."

*August 18*

"Benny calling. Do you want Barbara to come or not? I want to find out what you want me to do. Please give me a call Monday. Thank you."

*August 21*

"Hi, John. This is Benny calling. I'll be there Sunday, October fourteenth. Barbara will be there. OK? I'll repeat: Barbara will be there Sunday, October fourteenth. All right, bye."

Lisa said the primary objective of any cross-dressing support group is to assist the individual in knowing that he or she is part of a community.

"You are really creating a new person because you weren't raised as feminine," said Lisa. "The first thing is to get Ben to know that he's not alone, since most people do this alone at home. It usually begins at puberty around age twelve and then the question goes immediately to sexuality with 'Am I gay?' This is natural for the individual but not necessarily acceptable to others."

Prior to working with Ben, McClendon was aware for years of Ben's cross-dressing activities. She had heard through her professional network about "the guy that likes to sit on the front steps in panty hose."

"That's Ben trying to let people know about Barbara, but coming across as eccentric," explained Lisa.

Following the first meeting of ConnecticuTView, Lisa spoke with the RSG facilitator, Maureen Thomas, about Ben. Lisa wanted to offer reassuring messages about Ben's desires.

"If Ben is going to be a woman, she'll have to look like one and do the things that women do. If not, how can he feel the way a woman feels and be regarded as a woman by the people around him?" Lisa asked rhetorically.

Ben found the February cross-dressing support group meeting liberating and vividly recalled the moment when he was able to name the person he becomes when he cross-dresses. The naming experience allowed him to further develop the personality.

"Barbara is a good-looking girl. She has nice-looking legs," said Ben, describing his female creation. "She likes to stay in, but maybe later she can go out. She gets nervous going out. She's not used to going out."

"She's fifty-five years old and has an apartment in [my town]. She lives with me," said Ben. "She likes to watch TV but wants to go out, but I tell her she can't go out yet; it's not safe. She likes to clean the apartment."

Lisa said the first time she heard the name "Barbara" was at the February meeting. The group was hosting their annual tag sale where members can sell unwanted clothes and accessories. Ben was given a generous welcome.

"I gave [Ben] a blonde wig," said Lisa. "He was good at styling. He loved it and picked up a black evening gown that fit well. He looked cute and got lots of compliments. She was a happy girl. She was enthralled at being called 'Barbara' during that night and it harkens back to that moment when that woman inside is recognized by others as being good. It's very powerful."

The evening made an indelible impression on Ben. For the first time he was able to celebrate his desires around others who had similar feelings. The evening's activities assisted him with honing a wardrobe for Barbara by discovering the outfits that made her look good.

"She dresses in evening gowns, long wigs, medium heels, black tights, and purses," said Ben, describing Barbara's wardrobe. "She enjoys makeup and lipstick. She needs to learn how to use powder."

Barbara's transformation is not complete without her use of a feminine sanitary napkin. Just as Ben had to create the personality that came to be known as Barbara in a secret environment, wearing a sanitary napkin was one of the small but significant symbols that allowed him to celebrate his alter-ego in private. He said he has been doing this for years.

"It just sits in there toward the front. It's comfortable," said Ben. "It completes her."

Ben said his earliest memory of cross-dressing was as a ten-year-old. He said he stood on the kitchen table and served as the model when a family member sewed dresses. "I used to be the dummy," said Ben with a laugh. "I would stand on the kitchen table. I would stand there and she would pin the dress together."

Ben's childhood play activities did not include dressing up with friends. Cross-dressing has always been something he experienced alone. The clothes he used as a child were mostly borrowed from other family members, which included a favorite short dress and undergarments. Once dressed, he felt safe in his bedroom where he said he would "just hang around."

Ben has never appeared as Barbara in front of his friends or staff. The activity is so shrouded in conflicting emotions for Ben that he is even shy about presenting Barbara to McClendon. Through friendship and trust, McClendon said she wants Ben to know that Barbara can appear whenever she is around and that Barbara is safe in her presence. McClendon has been quick to understand the separateness of the two personalities and has helped Ben incorporate them both in their daily routine.

"Ben does not clean, Barbara cleans," said McClendon, observing that Ben and Barbara both exhibit traditional male-female domestic roles. "When the apartment needs to be cleaned, I have to tell Ben to ask Barbara to clean, and then it gets done. When I came in [this morning], Barbara was out with the mop scrubbing the kitchen floor."

McClendon said that within the first three months of working with Ben, she began to notice a pattern. McClendon said she knows whether Ben or Barbara will greet her for the day before entering the apartment. The self-conscious Barbara leaves the door unlocked, hides in the backroom or bathroom, and waits to be encouraged into the living room. Ben leaves the door locked.

"Ben gets nervous," said McClendon. "He's not fully comfortable having me see Barbara, but Barbara's out every time I come, unless we're going out. Ben has to get comfortable with Barbara."

As Ben became more comfortable discussing his cross-dressing activities and developing Barbara's personality, he began saying during the RSG meetings that he was gay, even though he had previously stated that he was heterosexual. No one ever challenged his declaration, but it was always thought that he was confusing sexuality with the desire to cross-dress. When questioned about whether he was gay, it was obvious that Ben was indeed confusing the two.

"I enjoy being with a woman more than a man," he clarified and added that he was confused by the terminology.

Ben identifies as a heterosexual man and says he is not uncomfortable being the only heterosexual member of the RSG. Until recently, he had a girlfriend who was also developmentally disabled, but she moved to another state to be with family and the two decided to end their relationship.

During the first interview for this profile, Ben wanted to appear as Barbara. Dressed in a smart-looking outfit—a below-the-knee gray skirt, white ruffled blouse, sheer black stockings, low heels, and a black wig—Barbara made a convincing feminine presentation. Assisting in the allure is Ben's smaller physique. At five-feet-seven-inches tall and 150 pounds, Ben has a frame that affords him an easy and convincing transition in contrast to other cross-dressing men who have bulkier frames.

Although Ben has a forty-five-year history of cross-dressing and wanted to show Barbara to me, the experience was still unsettling for him. Even in the comfortable surroundings of his own apartment, he sat in the corner of the sofa fidgeting with his wig and clothes.

Ben said he does not know why he likes to cross-dress, but when he does the experience makes him feel good about himself and relaxes him. He said he has never had a picture taken of himself dressed as a female and asked if I would take his picture in the interview. At the next RSG meeting when I gave him a copy of the photo, he was delighted with the image. He also called several times to ask if I would take Barbara's picture again since he purchased some new clothes.

## October 12, conversation

"That was the first time I've ever seen her. She looked pretty good, but she could do a better job with new clothes and a better wig," he said, excited to be discussing Barbara's pictures and wardrobe.

Ben asked if Barbara should come to the RSG open house on October 14, and I told him this was probably not the best time to bring Barbara. There would be other opportunities to introduce Barbara to the group.

"It needs to be safe; that's what staff keep telling me," said Ben.

## November 12, RSG meeting

I gave Ben a picture of Barbara that was taken during our interview. He was very pleased and had a huge smile on his face during the meeting. He kept it private, however, preferring not to share it with the other members. He asked if we could arrange another time when Barbara could have her picture taken in different clothes.

I told Ben we could take the photographs when we got together again.

## November 13, messages

Ben left three messages within one hour. He was excited about some of his new purchases for Barbara and wanted to have a picture of her in the new clothes:

First message: "Hi, John. This is Benny. Give me a call at my apartment. I'll be here for a while. Barbara wants to have her picture taken. She'll have a different dress on and a blonde wig. But give me a call. Leave it on my answering machine and I'll get back to you. OK, John? Thank you. Bye."

Second message: "Hi, John. This is Benny. Please give me a call because Barbara wants to know when you are coming to take her picture again. All right? I'll get back to you. Bye."

Third message: "Hi, John. This is Benny calling. The reason I'm calling is Barbara wants you to—I want you to call me back because

Barbara wants you to take a picture of her in her new dress and blonde wig. So please give me a call and let me know when you can do it. OK? Bye."

*November 13, conversation*

After three messages, I called Ben since it was obvious he was excited about his new purchases. He said he wanted additional photographs of Barbara taken in her new outfits—a blue evening dress, pink flat shoes, a couple of skirts, and a blonde wig.

I told him we could schedule an appointment after I returned from vacation the following week.

*November 14-15, three messages*

Ben called three times during these two days and left messages regarding the photographs as Barbara.

*November 19, telephone conversation with Maureen Thomas, RSG Facilitator*

I shared my concern with Maureen Thomas that Ben was continually calling to ask about having his picture taken as Barbara. I understood his excitement, but wanted to better understand his incessant calling and since she knew him better, hoped she could explain the behavior.

"As Ben has lost his girlfriend, he's gotten more into the cross-dressing," said Thomas, who added that Ben was looking for others to share in his cross-dressing activities. "It's going to be difficult for him to find a woman he can have an intimate relationship with who will be accepting of his cross-dressing activities. He's excited with his new identity and as he comes forward and has some acceptance he's running with it. You are someone he obviously trusts and feels safe in sharing this with you."

More than anyone in the Rainbow Support Group, Ben has had the most difficult time finding acceptance for his cross-dressing activities, not just from his support network but also from himself. Throughout his life, he has had to balance the desire to cross-dress with society's condemnation for doing so. The conflict has created tremendous turmoil in his life, yet he has been consistently creative in finding opportunities to experience the innate desire.

What has been fascinating to observe is that despite the absence of a tutor or even an understanding friend, he already knew about Barbara's existence. While other members of the group look for companionship or a partner as their primary interest, Ben's journey has been acutely focused on developing a relationship with his feminine personality. The challenge now is not in helping Ben accept Barbara, since that has already occurred. Rather, the challenge will be for those people who provide support to Ben—specifically his service providers, friends, and family—to accept Ben's decisions.

# Chapter 13

# Lisa

One of the saddest moments of my professional life occurred at 2:20 p.m. Friday, August 17, 2001.

I had a 2:00 appointment scheduled in my office with Mark (an alias), a public relations consultant who facilitates a cross-dressing support group at the NHGLCC. Mark was going to finish a discussion we started in May regarding Ben's participation in the group. Mark and I last spoke in May, when we arranged a concluding meeting, so I gave him a confirmation telephone call in the morning.

The first time I met Mark was during NHGLCC's festive and crowded holiday party in December 1999. Because he was dressed as his feminine alter ego, Lisa, and was introduced as a member of the ConnecticuTView support group for cross-dressers and their friends, I immediately asked Lisa to speak with Ben. They hit it off and made plans for Ben to attend one of the group's upcoming meetings.

During a few subsequent telephone calls over the next two years, I came to know Lisa and Mark only as Mark, and for our first visit he came to my office casually dressed as Mark. In addition, when we spoke just a few hours before this meeting he continued to speak with me as Mark.

Around 2:15 p.m. that day, I stepped out to the receptionist to ask if Mark had arrived. He hadn't. Since he was late, I returned to my office and became immediately involved in another project.

My phone rang five minutes later and the receptionist said in a matter-of-fact manner, "[There is a Lisa here] to see you."

Flustered and unable to recognize the name, I stalled for a moment. Suddenly a sense of horror flushed over me as I realized who was in the lobby. For all of my desire to be understanding and accepting of transgender people, my true feelings materialized in a flash and I was immobilized.

"Well, are you coming out or should I send her in?" the receptionist asked after the pause became awkward.

Standing up and straightening my clothes, I heard laughter and a buzz of whispers outside my office. My office is on a corner adjacent to a waiting area for client members and their staff returning from their work sites. The area usually begins filling up between 2:15 and 2:30 p.m. and today it was packed. As I emerged from my office, all conversation stopped—dead silence—when I called out to Lisa from across the room. She had started walking down a far hallway, which was toward the ladies' room, but I thought she was misdirected and was looking for my office.

Lisa walked through a gauntlet of staff, who remained silent as they tried to erase the smirks from their faces. Closing the door to my office behind us, I fumbled an attempt to begin the discussion.

"Were those people laughing at me?" Lisa asked. It was a question we both knew the answer to. To help us both save face and to manage my own discomfort, I told her that they were not laughing at her. I explained that the area is a waiting room and everyone was happily looking forward to the weekend, and so they were in good spirits.

At 200 pounds and six feet tall without heels, Lisa is a big girl. She does a good job of making an inconspicuous presentation, and on this visit she was appropriately dressed for a Friday afternoon. She wore a plain summer skirt, brown scoop-neck leotard top covering a large bosom, hoop earrings, a long auburn wig with bangs, and three-inch heels thick enough to support a Lane Bryant-like frame.

Her makeup was equally appropriate. It was not garishly applied like a drag queen ready for a glamorous evening, but subtle with just enough makeup and muted lipstick to cover a freshly shaven face. Even though Mark has obviously practiced his feminine persona and can pass undetected at first glance, everyone was aware of who had walked through the lobby that afternoon and, unfortunately, some staff members felt justified in making their reactions obvious.

The embarrassed and appalled feeling I felt when Lisa asked about the ridicule from staff was actually three separate and simultaneous emotions. I have spent the past twelve years at an employer whose primary mission is to provide support for people with disabilities. The hundreds of people who visit the agency every day come from many different backgrounds and cultures. Some are homeless, mentally ill, profoundly disfigured, or in need of personal care assistance.

Until that day, I had never witnessed an incident in which an individual was ridiculed for who he or she was or for appearance when entering the building—and certainly never in the person's presence. I felt more than anger or disappointment toward a group of college-educated staff who are supposed to display professional courtesies toward others. I felt emotionally betrayed by the people I work with, who are supposed to demonstrate professional behavior. The incident shook me to the core.

On further inspection of my feelings, I became aware that not all of the disappointment was directed toward a few naive young staff. Over the past two years of trying to connect Ben with ConnecticuTView, Mark and I had several conversations, both on the phone and in person, and I felt relaxed around him. Mark told me he identified as heterosexual, had a girlfriend, and had discovered that he lived about one-third of the time as Lisa.

I have great empathy for people who try to live an honest and open life. People who are transgender have few legal protections and are among the most maligned individuals, even within the gay community. Ironically, it was primarily transgender people who are credited with starting the modern gay movement during the Stonewall Inn rebellion against police bias in New York City's Greenwich Village in June 1969 (D'Emilio and Freedman, 1997). Cross-dressing, when not intended to be comedic, has elicited violent reactions from people who rigidly believe in gender roles.

When I invited Mark to visit, I expected him to arrive as his male persona, especially after having just confirmed the appointment with him a few hours earlier. When the receptionist called to announce Lisa's arrival, I paused at first to recall the name, since we did not have an appointment. I would have paused regardless of who called unexpectedly.

However, I cannot help thinking there was something more to the incident. In fact, I believe Mark had set me up. I can only imagine what Mark's feelings must be watching the reactions on unsuspecting faces as they figure out Lisa. Earlier in the year, Mark explained that he wanted to write a book similar to John Howard Griffin's *Black Like Me*, in which a white man undergoes a temporary skin darkening treatment to experience life as a black man. Mark wanted to legally become Lisa for one year and write about his experiences. He planned to get a job as Lisa, become a nonsexual friend to his girlfriend, and present himself to the community as Lisa both day and night. Mark was set to go before a judge the following week to discuss changing his name. I believe the few hours between my confirming phone conversation with Mark and Lisa's appearance in my office was not a whimsical change of plans which came over my guest, but rather a deliberate effort to record reactions as preparation for the book. Still, that does not excuse inappropriate behavior from people in a professional setting.

The third concern was my own reaction. Embarrassment and fear are the feelings I believe were present during the incident. I was partly embarrassed because I already knew what to expect of Lisa's appearance. Although she presents herself well, Lisa is still a trompe l'oeil, and I knew the ridicule being directed at her would soon transfer to me by association. The other times that I have been aware of being in the presence of transgender people, it has always been in the safety of gay settings where it is acceptable to pretend. The embarrassment I felt was that I, too, would be obligated to uphold a deception no one believed.

I am also disappointed with my own naiveté, for not realizing there is no sacred space for those who are different. But it was the fear I felt that has come to define the moment for me. The fear is that even with some legal and social protections for the cultural group I identify with, specifically the gay, lesbian, bisexual, and transgender community, somehow it is still acceptable for co-workers to mock me and my community members, even in our presence. The incident reminded me of junior and senior high school where I was verbally taunted and physically assaulted. The incident robbed me of the comfort to feel emotionally safe in my place of employment and to truly believe that my co-workers have exceptional manners and compassion for people who are different.

In an attempt to seek closure with my own feelings over this incident, I confronted the staff that I knew had laughed at Lisa. Only one individual apologized for the actions of the group. I accepted the apology. Surprisingly, it was liberating and allowed me to release some of the anger I felt at the injustice. As for the others who denied being involved, I take comfort in having at least confronted them. The exchange let them know everyone who enters the agency, regardless of how they are dressed or who they are, will be regarded with the respect and dignity that everyone deserves.

# SECTION III:
# THE LEADERS

# Chapter 14

# Facilitator, Maureen Thomas

"In many ways, it is like the 1950s in regards to sexuality. Our clientele are still treated as if they don't have a desire for intimacy," said Thomas, speaking of the period in the nation's history that was an antiseptic prelude to the sexual revolution. "It's still very much like that time."

The mark of a good support-group facilitator is someone who encourages participation from group members. Required skills include listening to the discussion, noticing patterns, guiding the topic, and assisting the participants to experience a sense of resolution.

With twenty-six years of experience working with people with developmental disabilities, Maureen Thomas's participation in the RSG was a welcome surprise. Her role as the group's facilitator evolved from being a casual observer to serving as the professional linchpin. Through her involvement, members are able to share their hopes and frustrations in a controlled and comfortable environment.

Thomas has a consistent and unassuming presence that seems to allow members to reveal what is going on inside of them. Through trust, she encourages them to speak about whatever is on their minds. With minimal words, she conveys an understanding that sexuality is a healthy component of being an adult.

There are multiple reasons that Thomas became an active member of the group. As the mother of a gay son, as a psychotherapist, and as a person who has had different sexual identities at different stages in her life, she is in a unique position not only to provide counseling for group participants but, equally important, to also counter the systemic homophobia and heterosexism prevalent throughout the human services profession.

In 1991, Connecticut became the third state in the country to offer civil rights protection for its gay and lesbian citizens (CWELF, 1995).

Agencies and state officials have a legal responsibility to respect sexual orientation issues in their workforce and client base. Thomas said that although the spirit of the law may be discussed by those at the top levels, when it comes to those providing direct care, personal biases often prevail in their relationship with clients.

"The reality is that is doesn't penetrate. It doesn't trickle down to the front line. Although it is a little bit better now compared to the recent past, there are still direct care staff that are real hard-line. Management may feel that they are supporting self-determination, but the reality is that it doesn't penetrate," said Thomas.

As someone who has spent her entire career working with DD/MR people in Connecticut, Thomas said that the profession has been slow to change.

"[A state agency] has many employees that are lifers that are not known for being progressive," she said, referring to employees who work their entire career with the state agency and also at private non-profit agencies.

"Some agencies can be progressive toward sexuality and some have a policy of no sexuality," she explained. "The truth is that clients do engage in sex and people know it, but they act as though as long as it stays underground, they won't have to get involved. No one wants to rock the boat."

Thomas said a generalized view of the human services profession is that staff enter the profession more as an altruistic career decision than for the monetary benefits offered. Although there is usually some truth in a stereotype, she feels that many job seekers settle for the profession when they are unable to secure more lucrative or accommodating positions in other fields. And since the human services field is in the business of supporting people who are different, she feels the profession has always provided a haven for gay employees as well as those who bring fundamental religious views to the job.

"You get quiet gays and noisy [religious fundamentalists]," she said with a chuckle, acknowledging a dichotomy in the rank-and-file workforce. "The gay people want to stay in the closet and the [religious] staff feel entitled to impose their beliefs on the clients. You can get people to mouth the words, to sound progressive, but direct care staff are still going to say what they want to clients when they are on their own. Their personal biases are going to surface, and yet they can have the greatest impact in the lives of the clients."

Thomas began her involvement in the Rainbow Support Group as a support for Ben. She was there to ensure the group was appropriate for Ben and also to observe his social interactions at the community center. Since then, she became the group's second and permanent facilitator because she has firsthand knowledge of the problems created when people with disabilities are denied the right to healthy sexual expression.

"I knew some agencies were heavy-handed in regards to sexuality," said Thomas, referring to the wide range of opinions on homosexuality at various agencies. "If the person was gay, then the staff would say, 'Oh, you really don't mean that,' and then try to set the person up in straight settings."

Thomas described a recent situation in which a staff member observed two women engaged in sexual activities at a group home. She said the staff person refused to accept that the two women were in love with each other.

"This is more the majority view because staff are expected to model and shape behavior," said Thomas. "The result is that you will get self-hating gay people [with DD/MR]. You see this mostly in institutional folks, but the irony is that gay sex is rampant. It is also severely punished and treated in a derisive manner."

Thomas recalled a series of events involving one of the state-run institutions that made an indelible impression on her at the beginning of her career. When men were caught engaging in same-sex sexual activities, they were punished by either having hot pepper powder sprinkled on their penis or placed in isolation for a period of time. She said that although current behavioral plans have advanced beyond such punitive conditions, the profession has not progressed far from such antiquated views of sexuality. There continues to be a pervasive expectation that as long as no one discusses sex or sexuality, hopefully the individuals with DD/MR will not be inclined to focus on it.

"In many ways, it is like the 1950s in regards to sexuality. Our clientele are still treated as if they don't have a desire for intimacy," said Thomas, speaking of the period in the nation's history that was an antiseptic prelude to the sexual revolution. "It's still very much like that time."

Thomas said that although sexuality and sexual expression are a basic human right, the profession has a responsibility to assist clients with having appropriate and healthy opportunities for intimacy. She referred to one example in which two men who lived in a group home and who were friends and wanted their relationship to become sexual became frustrated by a house rule that prohibited sexual activity. Although there may be good reasons for enforcing a no-sex policy in a group home, the men tried in vain to enlist the support of their residential staff to help them secure an alternate location and thus abide by the rule, since the only privacy they could experience occurred when no one was in their immediate vicinity for a few moments. The disregard by staff for the men's desire for intimacy manifested in each individual having numerous behavioral incidents that eventually severed their friendship.

"If people are not allowed privacy, how will they ever have a chance at intimacy with dignity?" Thomas asked. She added that opportunities for clients to clandestinely connect with their peers are decreasing as large institutions close. "As bad as the old training schools were with their harsh punishments, their residents had more opportunities to engage in sex than they do now in group homes."

During RSG meetings, Thomas has made it clear that members can discuss a broad range of topics. From current events to difficulties at work, to frustration over lack of privacy or independence, to dating, to sexual activities—all topics are appropriate when they are raised within the group.

"I do feel a strong motivation to help the members channel their desires into healthy behaviors so that they are not having sex with strangers; there is no exploitation, no unprotected sex, and no emotional toll on the members. An important function of the group is that this gives them another community to connect with and counter some of the negative messages they may have received from staff. It's a healthy forum to relate sexually with peers, and hopefully they can look within the group to settle with someone, or at least develop friends that feel as they do," she said.

Thomas made a comparison between watching her own son come out during high school and college in the mid-1990s and observing the members as they learn to accept their sexuality by participating in the RSG. She was aware that the maternal feelings she felt regarding her son's coming-out experience were similar to wanting to provide a safe and accepting environment where RSG members are free to explore their desires.

"As a mother, I recall watching my son manifesting his sexuality. Watching him come out was always fascinating. My son came out at sixteen," said Thomas, who acknowledged that her son at first tried to conform to the activities of his peers. "He dated girls and did the typical things kids do during those years to fit in."

Thomas said that just as her son found acceptance and felt empowered once he founded a gay-straight alliance (GSA) at a private high school, RSG members also developed stronger self-images once they began participating in the support group. She was concerned, because her son's coming-out experience occurred during the age of AIDS, but she was grateful to see his self-esteem blossom when he took on a leadership role in the GSA.

More than any other topic, members of the RSG discuss their desires for friendships and partners. Thomas said that although clients may desire intimate relationships, they are frequently not given the opportunity to develop the necessary skills to explore their sexuality or finesse courtships with interested partners. The dilemma is even more difficult for those who have more severe disabilities.

"Some clients are not able to handle a relationship," she said. "They may not be mature enough to sustain a long-term relationship since they have not been given the training or opportunity to practice having a real relationship."

Thomas said that if someone has a desire for sex, ignoring his or her wishes and impulses only contributes to unsafe behaviors. If someone has a desire for sex, no matter how diligently he or she is supervised, opportunities will arise. However, they may not be the safest opportunities and may leave the client vulnerable to assault, sexually transmitted diseases, and emotional stress.

"Mentally retarded people have a hard time with safe sex. They can easily get involved in unsafe situations and engage in risky behaviors," said Thomas, careful not to diminish the real dangers for people who live in a sheltered environment. "There are people out there that prey on gay men and on those that are perceived as vulnerable."

Thomas also said the human services profession needs to do more to assist staff and clients to better understand what constitutes competency and consent. She feels staff and management have an obligation to provide opportunities in which clients can experiment and act on their sexual desires.

"It can be hard for someone with mild MR to make distinctions between abuse and consensual sex," she said. "They may have second thoughts afterward, and that doesn't mean abuse. There may also be encouragement [from staff] to label consensual sex as abusive, because they may be embarrassed if caught or staff may be uncomfortable with their sexual activities."

One situation Thomas was called to evaluate involved two men who were having a sexual relationship. Staff were unsure whether the participation of both men, who were in their thirties, was mutual or if one had been coerced. The first man, who Thomas described as physically large, with autism and low-to-mild mental retardation, was infatuated with another man who had more severe retardation, was nonverbal, and was the size of an adolescent boy.

"Both seemed pleased with their relationship, but the whole legal system and reporting requirements kicked in," said Thomas, who was perplexed over how best to determine whether their relationship had mutual consent. "How can [the nonverbal man] show competency and make a decision? Just his actions would seem to be a suitable indication of his desire."

Thomas said that the nonverbal man was known to enjoy giving men hugs and it seemed that he was not objecting to the relationship. When Thomas interviewed the larger man, he told her he enjoyed having a young male in his bed and that he was comforted at night by having a young companion next to him.

"He probably did have other boys in his bed when he was growing up in the institution," said Thomas. "That was his comfort and his affection. In my heart, I wanted to leave them alone, but legally there was no way I could say the severely retarded man was competent to make those decisions. And that left the agency vulnerable."

The solution came when the agency got the larger man a huge teddy bear that was nearly the same size as the other man. The substitution seemed to satisfy his desire to hold onto something during the night.

"Ideally, I wish he would be able to meet someone like himself and they could be in an apartment where there was no third shift and let nature take its course, but that's not the case," said Thomas, who felt the agency and staff would be vulnerable if something unfortunate happened. "This seems to give him comfort and until he can find someone, thankfully, this seems to be solving the problem."

Thomas said that clients often receive many conflicting messages from staff regarding sexual activity. The situation is most restrictive for those who live in a group home with many different staff providing daily supervision or for those adult children who still live with parents or family members with strict house rules. In the confusion, clients may continue to pursue infatuations or sexual activities, while simultaneously attempting to hide their desires or behaviors if they believe their staff is uncomfortable with same-sex activities.

"For example, [one member of the RSG who lives in a group home] wants to have gay sex, but since he is not his own guardian and his family is not supportive, he is not allowed to get involved with anyone," said Thomas, who added that she has firsthand experience with staff writing behavioral plans that attempt to conform the behavior of GLBT clients to heterosexual mores.

"There is such a variety of opinions on sex and sexuality and it doesn't translate down," said Thomas, who feels that many more clients would be inclined to identify with the GLBT community if they were given more freedom to explore their sexuality. "You can intervene if someone says, 'Please help me,' but if not, you can't intervene."

Based on her professional observations, Thomas compared the sexual behaviors and identities of fifty- to eighty-year-old clients who grew up in institutions with twenty- to forty-year-old clients who grew up in group homes.

"My clinical experience has been that eighty percent of men I have seen that are now fifty to eighty years old, who are now dying out, are inclined toward homosexual behavior," she said, careful to distinguish between behavior and orientation. "I wouldn't call it gay identity, but it is definitely gay behavior and arousal."

From the 1940s to the 1970s, Connecticut maintained two large institutions where thousands of state residents with DD/MR lived, one of which is still operating in a limited capacity. Thomas said that since the institutions were segregated by gender, the only opportunities for intimacy were clandestine and with others of the same sex. In addition, the state-supported residences were notoriously understaffed, with ratios of one staff member to thirty clients, which allowed clients more opportunities to connect with one another, especially when compared to the current staffing requirements in residences supported by private nonprofit agencies of one or two staff members for six clients. Thomas said that during the prior arrangements, sexual activity was common, usually went unreported, and was predominately within the same gender.

"The men that spent their critical sexual years, from adolescence to early adult, in the institution segregated by gender were conditioned for same-sex arousal," she said. "Now, with the younger men and women in our group homes, they don't have those same experiences and you can speculate that those who prefer same-sex partners have a biological orientation toward homosexuality."

Thomas spoke about one young man in his twenties with mental retardation and an androgynous personality. She said the man grew up in a heterosexual household and had numerous coeducational socializing opportunities. Since he was encouraged to make his own decisions, he declared his homosexuality as an adolescent.

"No one tried to push him into any path," said Thomas. "This is his nature surfacing, which is definitely gay."

# Chapter 15

# Founder, John D. Allen

"Immediately after heading upstairs to the dance floor, I bought a beer and saw Keith standing off to the side. Wasting no time, I asked him to dance, we exchanged numbers, and our courtship began. Aside from a few indiscretions early on, most of my gay life has revolved around a monogamous relationship with my partner. It is a life I would choose again."

The earliest memory I have of a gay experience was during the second grade. I was sitting in the backyard at my best friend's house after school talking about our new gym teacher. The still-vivid memory occurred just a few days into the new school year and involved a beautiful, sunny September afternoon. We sat cross-legged on the back lawn, plucking wide blades of grass and positioning them between our thumbs to make whistles. We had a big topic to discuss— Mr. Kepple. My recollection of the conversation was that we pored over his muscles, the tufts of hair popping up over his tight T-shirt, and his manly good looks. We pondered the games he would have for us that year, the whistle dangling from his neck, and most definitely what he looked like in his underwear. It would take nearly another twenty years before I had enough self-awareness to begin a new identity and act on my sexuality.

Most gay people have a coming-out story, and listening to others reveal their story is a particularly favorite pastime of mine. My own story, which I like to trot out whenever conversations steer toward the subject, occurred the first time I mustered the courage to go into a gay disco bar. It was March 6, 1982—the night I met my partner, Keith. In a last-minute internal conflict, I walked around the block a few times before sheepishly going inside. The air was thick with smoke and sweat. I felt light-headed with both fear and exhilaration. The room was packed with men and for the first time I saw them not as forbidden fruit, but possibilities. Immediately after heading upstairs to the dance floor, I bought a beer and then saw Keith standing off to the side. Wasting no time, I asked him to dance, we exchanged numbers, and our courtship began. Aside from a few indiscretions early on, most of my gay life has revolved around a monogamous relationship with my partner. It is a life I would choose again.

Although that is the story I use to mark my gay awakening, there are also many other notable events in my coming-out continuum. Coming out is not just a one-time event, since gay people must decide whether to reveal their sexual orientation every time they begin a new social interaction (Savin-Williams, 2001). Gay people must continually make this decision in their daily conversations with professional colleagues or social exchanges with strangers and acquaintances simply because personal anecdotes surface in routine conversations. Some of my other significant coming-out stories involve the moments I told each of my siblings, my parents, employer, and the greater community through the regional daily newspaper. Each event was a new forum that allowed me to validate my feelings and rebuild my life from a previously hidden gay perspective.

Coming out is a very deliberate activity that, no matter how many times it occurs, requires a conscious pause before proceeding. Society is heterosexually oriented—it validates conformity and demonizes nonconformity. Throughout high school, college, and early adulthood, I tried desperately to conform by dating women, seeking approval from others for my decisions, and starting life paths that were not comfortable. Not until my life had become miserable, trapped in a heterosexual lie, was I willing to risk everything—family, friends, job—to become reborn. The journey did not take one night, but rather it took years for me to become comfortable with my new consciousness.

It is a misnomer that gay men dislike women. On the contrary, I have had wonderful experiences with women and cherish the sexual sharing and experimentation I enjoyed with some of my female partners. However, there was always the realization that the sex was incomplete and that I felt like an imposter in the relationship. Although I feel fortunate to have avoided heterosexual marriage and thereby spared both of us the agony of certain frustration, I also look back with fondness at my sexual memories that include women.

My partner and I are both very fortunate to have come from loving, stable homes with parents who were married for more than fifty years. We are both one of five children, the middle child and the eldest son, and we both were named for our fathers. We also have similar coming-out stories. Although our families initially offered only tepid support for our nonmainstream sexuality, neither of us was rejected or excluded from family functions. In fact, as our partnership grew, our families quickly came to regard us as a couple. I am especially forgiving of their initial responses since our coming-out experiences occurred prior to what I call the "Age of Ellen," before Ellen DeGeneres came out as a lesbian in her personal life and as her television character, and gay issues exploded into the national consciousness. Life for gay people is much better post-Ellen than before. As a gay activist who hears tragic tales from many gay people in the community, I realize both Keith and I were lucky to be born and raised by our families of origin.

Aside from being gay, I feel my life is pretty much like any other suburban, college-educated, partnered taxpayer. We live in a ranch house on a one-and-one-half-acre wooded lot in a beach community two blocks from Long Island Sound. My parents and brothers live in adjacent towns. I drive a pickup truck and over the past few years have enjoyed hanging out with my buddies down at the town dump and recycling center where I take leaves and branches in what has become a Saturday-morning ritual. For our twentieth anniversary, Keith and I adopted Nacho, a one-year-old, six-pound Chihuahua from an animal rescue agency, and now we cannot imagine life without him. We enjoy our home and have worked hard to make it cozy with plenty of domestic conveniences.

Keith and I never had a marriage or commitment ceremony. Our reason was that we would rather have nothing than participate in an event that does not offer the same benefits as heterosexual marriage. Nowhere in the country can gay people legally marry. Only in Vermont can gay couples establish a legal civil union that mirrors many of the same rights and privileges offered heterosexual couples, but the union is valid only in Vermont. On July 10, 2000, ten days after Vermont became the first state to offer the closest thing to gay marriage, we traveled to Vermont and participated in a double civil ceremony. We were the twenty-ninth couple to have a civil union in Brattleboro, and although the ceremony was personally significant, mostly for the opportunity to be part of gay history, the memory also has a dark side for our families.

Also present for the double civil union was my sister and her same-sex partner of twelve years, their six-year-old son, and my mother. Unbelievably, just two months after the ceremony, the relationship dissolved after my sister's partner left her to begin another relationship. Complicating the breakup is that their child was deliberately conceived, through donor insemination, by Keith and my sister's partner. Although our partners provided a biological origin, the two moms were the parents. As magically as our blended family began, once the breakup occurred we were all stunned to observe firsthand why gay families need the same legal protections as heterosexually headed families. Without a legal system to serve as chaperone and provide for a fair exit, the separation has become the most tragic divorce I have known.

The activist label is not one I usually use for myself, but others have used it to describe me to the media. In my youth, the turmoil I experienced attempting to conform instead of celebrating my gayness produced a quiet and lonely existence. I spent so much time trying to fit in and seek friendships with people that never materialized, that I focused little on the outside world. In retrospect, those years spent immobilized and floundering have now become my antithesis for how to live life. Gay issues are only some of the subjects in which I have a passionate interest. It is easy to focus on gay causes, in part, because there is such a great need to counter the misinformation about the gay community. With such a dearth of gay people willing to serve in leadership roles, I feel I am in a good place to be public with my life and the best resource available to any gay person to sway tenacious stereotypes is to simply live openly and deliberately.

As a part-time journalist and contributor to several regional publications, writing has become a powerful vehicle for me to impact my community. It was during graduate school when I realized I had a proficiency to write better than I spoke. At first writing only term papers, I also began writing press releases for some of my favorite groups, which led to writing for gay publications as a local reporter, and then writing for a chain of weekly, suburban newspapers. Writing has become a passion, and I take great joy in trying to build on each success in this newly discovered skill.

A writing project that has become a signature piece for me evolved from my master's thesis in urban studies at Southern Connecticut State University. The subject was a needs assessment of the gay community in southern Connecticut—New Haven is a city of 130,000 people and includes a metropolitan region of 250,000—which until that time was disconnected and invisible. My two-part project was to quantify the gay community and determine whether there was interest in supporting a GLBT community center. The results of the survey made front-page news in the fall of 1995. What emerged was a vibrant community of forty gay and gay-friendly groups, with combined memberships of 1,700 people and annual budgets totaling $2.3 million. Equally exciting, the respondents were unanimously supportive of creating a community center/centralized queer space where they could hold meetings, social events, and political activities.

Armed with this information, I began working on a ten-point marketing plan to establish the framework for a nonprofit agency, raise funds, and meet with key leaders in the region including politicians, business directors, and major media directors. I met with more than two dozen leaders in a nine-month span. The last meeting was with New Haven's mayor, John DeStefano, who was satisfied with what had been accomplished and who assisted our newly established board of directors in securing office space in one of the city's flagship locations. On November 18, 1996, what began as a graduate project became the first gay center in the city, the third gay center in Connecticut, and the seventy-sixth gay center in the country. The New Haven Gay & Lesbian Community Center has evolved into a true community resource that now serves as home to dozens of groups and events, including the unprecedented Rainbow Support Group.

Like my father and grandfather, I have been in professional sales my entire career. The first half of my career was spent selling industrial products in the Northeast until I felt drawn to find more altruistic employment. Around the same time, I also became less guarded in censoring myself at work, which proved to be incompatible with my employer at the time. It was in May 1987 when I traveled with a senior official on a West Coast trip to visit clients. I will never forget the grilling I received during one dinner with this senior employee regarding who I was dating, my plans for a family, and my life goals. I felt I had deftly and truthfully maneuvered the conversation without betraying my new gay identity. A week later at 4:30 p.m., I was asked to leave, told only, "You have no future here." Although I too knew I had no future there and was soon glad to be separated from such a good-ole-boy corporation where the men had their offices on the second floor, the women were all secretaries relegated to the first floor, and heterosexuality was a career requirement, there was great pain in being dismissed for who you are instead of your performance.

Most GLBT people I encounter include painful moments of being bullied, harassed, or worse in their personal histories. For me, one unforgettable incident occurred in the fall of 1973 when I was a junior in high school. My father's job brought us from Southern California to what was a quintessential New England town. I was painfully shy. There were no gay role models for me as a teen. I would eventually come out ten years later only when I had the safety of my own self-worth for support.

As painful as it is to admit, at various times growing up, I was fodder for bullies. On a fateful fall afternoon, I was sitting around the lunch table with friends when it started. I was caught off guard when I first heard my name. Horrifying and surreal, I heard it called out several times before I could pinpoint the direction of the voices. Slowly building, it grew from a single shout into a group chant—like a football team gang bang—with player after player pounding their fists in unison on the table: "John Allen is a faggot."

That image continues to haunt me. Wounded and humiliated, I wanted to die right then and there and immediately hated myself for being the sissy, the one singled out by a group of jocks and publicly ridiculed for being different. But how did it happen? I never did anything to those kids and most of them never knew me.

The only answer I can piece together over the years has been in knowing that the lead instigator of that infamous day, the one who chanted the loudest and the only one I remember from the crowd, would later turn out to be a well-known community theater actor. I still find it uncanny that this local thespian saw what would take me ten more years to figure out. He knew I was queer, and to be queer in 1973 was to be hated, ridiculed, and despised.

Often I have thought about the motivation behind my desire to speak publicly on sensitive gay issues. Certainly, I have enjoyed the spotlight that comes with being a representative for a community, but I also feel that I was well prepared for the role and accepted the responsibility with best intentions. I find it no coincidence that my professional and public coming out coincided with my employment at an agency that supports people with disabilities.

Working as an advocate for people with disabilities provided the emotional bridge for me to begin challenging the injustices I feel every day as an openly gay man, but it has not been without a personal cost. Although difficult to prove, I feel that being so public with my achievements on behalf of the gay community, and thereby acknowledging my sexuality, has hindered my career, even in a state that has gay civil rights protections (Woods, 1993). For all of the progress of the gay movement in recent years, my personal experience has revealed that any reference to sexuality in the workforce, especially in a profession that relies on public funds, has been a career liability.

As I survey the experiences of my gay life, I generally feel fortunate to have reached this point and in this condition. I have good health, a long-term partnership, a comfortable home, and the ability to enjoy my personal and financial resources. Even the tragedies of my past, from the mundane to the catastrophic, have provided important lessons and opportunities for growth. Focusing on the future, I feel a debt to my community to make gay life a more fulfilling experience for those who are perhaps unable to openly declare their sexuality. My attention is now directed toward facilitating a voice for gay, lesbian, bisexual, and transgender people with developmental disabilities and mental retardation, who are among the most maligned people in society. Truly, some of the greatest moments for me have been my efforts to normalize gay life and realize the power that all of us have to affect the world.

# Conclusion

When promoting any group, I have always believed in the motto, "Any press is good press," regardless of whether it includes bad news. Getting media coverage is critical to broadcasting a message. However, early in the process of spreading the word about the RSG, I came face to face with such a dilemma. Pushing for an interview with one of the prominent gay publications in New England, imagine my surprise and subsequent horror when the following headline appeared:

> A group nobody wanted to talk about: Being mentally disabled and gay was to admit what was once taboo—the developmentally disabled want sex. (*Bay Windows,* February 10, 2000)

The word *sex* screamed from the page. All I saw in the headline was that DD/MR people just want to have sex. I was furious that a copy editor had whittled the message of the RSG into something base. I thought the group was offering people freedom of expression. Of course sex was part of it, but it was more about providing a place where people who are supervised, controlled, and restricted— some for twenty-four hours a day—can have access to their feelings. The RSG is not just about sex. At its core, it is about changing the way society and the human services profession disallow people with intellectual disabilities the freedom to be honest about what is going on inside of them.

Once my surprise at seeing the headline subsided, I realized the truth in the message. The RSG *is* about sex. But more important, it is about providing a safe and healthy environment where people who think and feel the same way can meet, socialize, and consider the possibilities of forming emotional attachments that may ultimately lead to sex.

Many communities exist because of sex and sexual desire. Even in restrictive communities such as religious congregations, people who share similar feelings gather together, partner, and can choose to engage in sex. Unfortunately, this is not so for people with DD/MR—they have been de-sexed. They are denied the same opportunities because they are perceived as damaged people who are trapped forever in a childlike state—and children are to be protected from adult experiences. However, the need for sex is universal and the message of the RSG is that this community of adults has a right to love, to form relationships, and to enjoy their innate desires for sexual expression.

Staff members continually approach me to privately discuss clients who they feel are gay, yet are unacknowledged. One staff person relayed a story about a male client who regularly revealed his sexuality to anyone who paid attention.

The client, who had always lived at home, had led a sheltered life. The staff felt intimidated about discussing the subject of the RSG or sexuality in general, since the client's parents were devout practicing Roman Catholics, members of a church that has a strict policy on homosexuality. Since sexuality is not part of a vocational program, the staff members never raised the subject and, instead, focused only on the client's vocational program.

"He expresses his [gay] feelings at least once a week," said a staff person. "He brings in bodybuilding pictures, and when he sees a good-looking male in a magazine, he always makes a comment. He never discusses a girlfriend or even an interest in girls, but will make a side gesture if he notices a handsome man."

The staff person reported that during a renovation to his agency's building, the client was part of a landscaping crew working near the construction site. In one telling instance, the client was observed staring at a muscular construction worker, and before rejoining the crew he shook his hand in a gesture intimating that the worker was "hot."

"He was checking him out and made a hand gesture like he was a hot guy," the staff person said. "He's in his fifties and probably won't be able to act on his sexuality until he moves out of his folks' house, or else they die and he can live on his own."

The staff member said that although the client always maintains professional boundaries and does not touch other men, he continually demonstrates that he has a sexuality, is sexually aware, and has same-sex attractions. "Most staff are oblivious to the cues he gives about what is really going on within him," said the staff person.

Not allowing people to have appropriate sexual outlets can contribute to pathological behavior in some clients. For example, taking money away from a client who cross-dresses simply because a staff person is uncomfortable with the activity can be a contributing factor to the individual shoplifting. Similarly, when another client sneaks off to have unsafe sex because he or she feels forced to hide, the profession does a disservice to the people they serve. No matter what level of functioning clients have, and regardless of their disabilities, clients still get a message that gay sexual behavior is taboo. The hope for the profession is to create positive, healthy environments in which people with DD/MR are allowed the opportunity to experience a full range of human emotions. It is more than just sex; it is about acknowledging a personal truth.

Similarly, there may be gay staff who are sympathetic to the RSG and its mission but feel too intimidated to be openly supportive of the group and gay clients within their agency. The RSG is not simply helping to provide a place for people with DD/MR, it also serves as an advocacy resource for the entire human services profession. Such an experience occurred with an administrator, new to her agency, who said that she wanted to support the group as a volunteer and requested information. After I faxed a meeting announcement, she called to complain that I had breached a confidence with her, even though she was the one who requested the information. She said she was unaware that the literature, a one-page flyer that announced meeting dates, would contain the words *gay, lesbian, bisexual,* and *transgender.*

"Don't ever send a fax to me here again," she said, frightened, angry, and letting me know she was not out at work. "I can't afford to risk this getting around."

I explained that several people at her agency have already been sent information on the RSG, including the executive director, and that Connecticut passed a civil rights law protecting gay people from employment discrimination. I believe she felt that by receiving a flyer for a gay support group, she too would be labeled a lesbian by association.

"This turned out OK, because someone covered for me, but don't send me any more information," she said, closing the conversation.

The most powerful resource the gay community can use in the struggle for equality is a simple but deeply personal action. It is to come out. The only choice gay people have to make is whether to be honest with themselves. Those that are able to make the crossover can experience the satisfaction of correcting an imbalance. Unfortunately, the journey to come out can be too difficult for some to acknowledge, relegating the person to a life of unanswered questions.

Those who have found the RSG are the lucky ones, myself included. They have completed a journey and are comfortable with their decision to be true to their feelings. As human services professionals, there is an obligation to help people experience a life full of opportunities. Hopefully, that includes a level of comfort with their sexuality, the freedom to form intimate relationships, and opportunities to enjoy the wonder of sexuality.

# References

Bernstein, R.A. (1995). *Straight parents, gay children: Keeping families together.* New York: Thunder's Mouth Press.

Blumenfeld, W.J. (Ed.) (1992). *Homophobia: How we all pay the price.* Boston: Beacon Press.

Connecticut Women's Education and Legal Fund, Inc. (CWELF). (1995). *The legal rights of lesbians and gay men in Connecticut.* Hartford, CT: Author.

D'Emilio, J. and Freedman, E.B. (1997). *Intimate matters: A history of sexuality in America.* Chicago: University of Chicago Press.

Gay & Lesbian Alliance Against Defamation. (GLAAD). (2001). *Lesbian, gay, bisexual and transgender media reference guide.* New York: Author.

Hingsburger, D. (1991). *I contact: Sexuality and people with developmental disabilities.* Mountville, PA: VIDA Publishing.

Kempton, W. (1998). *Sex education for persons with disabilities that hinder learning: A teacher's guide.* Santa Barbara, CA: James Stanfield Company.

Ladew, D.P. (1998). *How to supervise people: Techniques for getting results through others.* Shawnee Mission, KS: National Press Publications.

Marcus, E. (1993). *Is it a choice? Answers to 300 of the most frequently asked questions about gays and lesbians.* New York: HarperCollins.

Monat-Haller, R.K. (1992). *Understanding & expressing sexuality: Responsible choices for individuals with developmental disabilities.* Baltimore: Paul H. Brookes.

Savin-Williams, R.C. (2001). *Mom, Dad, I'm gay. How families negotiate coming out.* Washington, DC: American Psychological Association.

The Arc (1982). Introduction to mental retardation. Available online: <http://www.thearc.org/faqs/mrqa.html>.

Woods, J.D. (1993). *The corporate closet: The professional lives of gay men in America.* New York: Free Press.